HYPERTENSION AND DYSLIPIDEMIA MANAGEMENT ESSENTIALS

Robert Miller Guthrie, MD

Professor of Emergency Medicine, Internal Medicine, and Pharmacology
Associate Director of Clinical Pharmacology
Ohio State University
Columbus, OH

2010

PHYSICIANS' PRESS
A DIVISION OF JONES AND BARTLETT PUBLISHERS
Sudbury, Massachusetts
BOSTON TORONTO LONDON SINGAPORE

World Headquarters
Jones and Bartlett Publishers
40 Tall Pine Drive
Sudbury, MA 01776
978-443-5000
info@jbpub.com
www.jbpub.com

Jones and Bartlett Publishers
Canada
6339 Ormindale Way
Mississauga, Ontario L5V 1J2
Canada

Jones and Bartlett Publishers
International
Barb House, Barb Mews
London W6 7PA
United Kingdom

Jones and Bartlett's books and products are available through most bookstores and online booksellers. To contact Jones and Bartlett Publishers directly, call 800-832-0034, fax 978-443-8000, or visit our website www.jbpub.com.

Substantial discounts on bulk quantities of Jones and Bartlett's publications are available to corporations, professional associations, and other qualified organizations. For details and specific discount information, contact the special sales department at Jones and Bartlett via the above contact information or send an email to specialsales@jbpub.com.

Production Credits
Senior Acquisitions Editor: Alison Hankey
Senior Editorial Assistant: Jessica Acox
Production Director: Amy Rose
Production Assistant: Laura Almozara
Senior Marketing Manager: Barb Bartoszek
V.P., Manufacturing and Inventory Control: Therese Connell
Composition: diacriTech, Chennai, India
Cover Design: Kate Ternullo
Cover Image: © MedicalRF.com/age fotostock
Printing and Binding: Cenveo
Cover Printing: Cenveo

Library of Congress Cataloging-in-Publication Data
Guthrie, Robert M.
Hypertension and dyslipidemia management essentials / Robert Miller Guthrie.
p. ; cm.
Includes bibliographical references and index.
ISBN-13: 978-0-7637-5926-1 (alk. paper)
ISBN-10: 0-7637-5926-0 (alk. paper)
1. Hypertension–Chemotherapy. 2. Hypotensive agents. 3. Lipids–Metabolism–Disorders–Chemotherapy. 4. Antilipemic agents. 5. Hyperlipidemia–Chemotherapy. I. Title.
[DNLM: 1. Hypertension–drug therapy. 2. Dyslipidemias–drug therapy. WG 340 G984h 2010]
RC685.H8G88 2010
616.1'32061–dc22

2009007867

6048
Printed in the United States of America
13 12 11 10 09 10 9 8 7 6 5 4 3 2 1

ABOUT THE AUTHOR

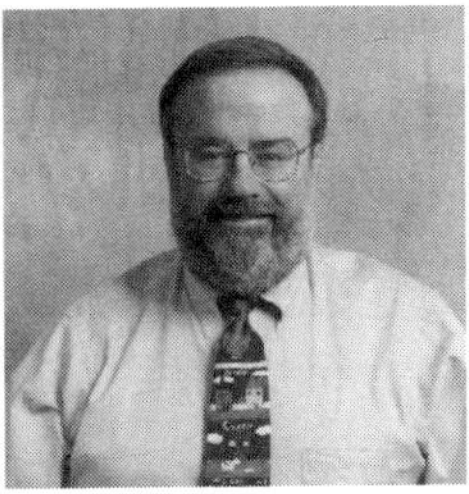

The son and grandson of physicians, Robert Miller Guthrie, MD, is a professor at Ohio State University. He received his bachelor's degree from the College of Wooster in Wooster, Ohio, and his medical degree from the University of Maryland. Dr. Guthrie is board certified in family medicine and internal medicine. He joined the faculty at Ohio State University in 1982.

At Ohio State, Dr. Guthrie conducts a research program evaluating new medications being developed for the US market. He has conducted over 65 such projects, and many of the medications that he has evaluated are currently used widely in the United States. Dr. Guthrie has published extensively, having authored over 60 peer-reviewed manuscripts, along with numerous abstracts and other papers. He has been a very active national speaker for physician education programs, with the goal of explaining the complicated emerging scientific data in a practical and usable format for practitioners.

TABLE OF CONTENTS

INTRODUCTION

Cardiovascular disease continues to be the leading cause of death in the United States and throughout the industrialized world.[1] Indeed, in the United States from 1900 until the present, except for the severe flu epidemic in 1918, heart disease has consistently been the leading cause of mortality year after year. In 2004, the year most recent statistics are available, cardiovascular disease, including all forms of heart and cerebrovascular disease, accounted for 2.4 million deaths. The second leading cause of deaths, cancer, was far behind at 550,000 deaths. In contrast, breast cancer accounted for only 41,000 female deaths, and HIV/AIDS only 13,000 deaths in both genders. Indeed, only 1 in 30 female deaths are from breast cancer, while 1 in 6 female deaths are from heart disease. Moreover, 1 in 2.6 deaths overall in both genders are from cardiovascular disease.[1]

Historically, deaths from cardiovascular disease rose dramatically and consistently through the early decades of the 20th century.[1] However, in the early 1970s this trend began to reverse, and there has been a gradual reduction in the rate of death from cardiovascular disease since then.[1] This new pattern has led to a dramatic drop in the overall incidence of cardiovascular disease and mortality over the last 35 years.[1] The reduction has been documented in a number of studies that also shed light on the factors producing this decline.

The Framingham Heart Study documents the reduction most clearly.[2] When the Framingham study compared the time periods of 1990–1999 with the original time period of 1950–1969, they found that mortality rates for coronary heart disease (CHD) had fallen by 59%, while the rates of sudden cardiac death had fallen by 49%. These reductions were seen across all patient groups, including those without previous CHD (nonsudden death down 74%) or those with prior CHD (nonsudden death down 62%).[2] Death rates declined 63% in men and 62% in women.[2]

The Framingham study noted that various cardiac risk factors, including systolic blood pressure, cholesterol, and smoking, had improved during these time frames. They also noted that the mortality improvements had occurred equally in smokers and nonsmokers.[2]

Other authors have noted and evaluated these patterns. Ford et al., looked at the decline in US CHD mortality rates between 1980 and 2000.[3] During this two-decade period, CHD deaths fell by nearly 50%. The authors calculated that 47% of the improvement was produced by treatments, like the management of acute myocardial infarction (MI) and heart failure, while 44% was due to risk factor reductions. However, in the risk factor reduction group, most of the benefit was from reductions in blood pressure and cholesterol, which are almost exclusively due to medication therapy.[3] The true lifestyle reductions of increased activity and smoking reduction are nearly offset by increases in weight and diabetes mellitus.[3] Therefore, the true reductions are produced by improvement in medical therapy.[4] Essentially, proper medication for the management of hypertension and high cholesterol have a clear record of reducing the death rate from stroke and heart attack by about 50% over the last 35 years.

The same pattern of a dramatic decline in the CHD deaths rates has been documented in other industrialized nations. In Finland, CHD deaths declined 63% between 1982 and 1997, with much of this reduction attributed to a reduction in cholesterol levels and somewhat less attributed to a reduction in blood pressure.[5] In Britain, there has been a 62% decline in MI between 1978 and 2004.[6] Much of this reduction is also attributed to reductions in cholesterol and blood pressure, emphasizing our need to continue to increase our efforts to prevent CHD through aggressive management of blood pressure and cholesterol.[7]

However, there are suggestions that we may be beginning to see a lessening, or even a cessation, of this pattern of dramatic reductions in CHD deaths. Recent autopsy data from Olmstead County, Minnesota, found that the decline in the severity of coronary artery disease had ceased in the years between 1995 and 2000.[8] This study is of course limited to 1 particular county, but it is concerning that, possibly secondary to the recent increase in obesity and diabetes mellitus, we may not continue to see continual improvement in CHD mortality in the future.[9]

Therefore, I have written this book to assist clinicians in the treatment of hypertension and high cholesterol, the 2 most easily-diagnosed, treatable risk factors for cardiovascular disease. As practitioners, we all must redouble our efforts to diagnose and then comprehensively manage these twin CHD risk factors, hypertension and elevated cholesterol.

Section 1

Hypertension

Chapter 1

Hypertension

EPIDEMIOLOGY AND IMPACT

Hypertension has become, and will likely remain, the ultimate primary care disorder of adults. It is diagnosed by simple measurements in the practitioner's office, and all subsequent evaluations, along with the treatment, are office-based procedures. Indeed, it remains an outpatient disorder especially if our management is successful in preventing the many cardiovascular events, like myocardial infarction, stroke, or heart failure, that result from uncontrolled blood pressure.

It comes as a shock to many practitioners that interest in treating stage I and stage II hypertension ("mild" and "moderate" in the old classification) only dates to 1970, within a month of my entry into medical school. The first treatment study of hypertension, in 1967, was an active treatment versus placebo study in patients with diastolic blood pressure (DBP) between 115 and 129 mm Hg, levels that today would be considered severe hypertension.[10] In 1970 the first effort to evaluate the treatment of lower DBP in the range of 95 to 110 mm Hg was published, showing dramatic reductions in stroke and heart failure.[11]

A series of other treatment trials followed, leading to a recognition of the importance of treating hypertension.[12] These trials, taken as a whole, showed that reducing blood pressure for as brief a period as 2 to 3 years could reduce stroke rates by 35% to 40% and coronary heart disease rates by 20% to 25%.[12]

Long-term studies illustrate the tremendous overall impact of this most common disorder. The Framingham Heart Study shows that nearly 90% of adults in the 55 to 65 age range will become hypertensive in their lifetime.[13] Since the crucial initial treatment article was published in 1970, we have seen slow but significant progress in identifying and treating patients with hypertension.

As our understanding of the impact of hypertension evolved over time, new questions arose and were answered. While the original research had focused on the treatment of elevated DBP, the question as to whether and how we should manage isolated systolic hypertension in the elderly was not answered until 1991. Using a diuretic-based regimen, the Systolic Hypertension in the Elderly Program showed that lowering an isolated systolic pressure reduced stroke, myocardial infarction (MI), and heart failure.[14] A subsequent European study (Systolic Hypertension in Europe—Syst-Eur) found similar results with a calcium channel blocker (CCB) and a regimen based on an angiotensin-converting enzyme inhibitor (ACE inhibitor).[15]

While the early trials conducted in the 1970s and 1980s had documented the importance of controlling hypertension in middle-aged adults in the industrialized world, the previously mentioned trials in the elderly presented strong evidence for the benefit of extending hypertension treatment to the elderly.[16] Recent research has shown the benefit of treating hypertension even in the *very elderly*, those above 80 years of age.[17] Indeed, in evaluating hypertension around the world, research shows that elevated blood pressure produces the same degree of increase in risk for cardiovascular events throughout the world.[18]

HYPERTENSION MANAGEMENT

As the focus of this book is the *management* of hypertension and hypercholesterolemia, we all need to clearly understand that hypertension and hypercholesterolemia are just part of the spectrum of conditions that increase the risk of cardiovascular disease. While hypertension and hypercholesterolemia are the 2 most directly diagnosed risk factors for the development of cardiovascular disease, the interrelation of those factors with many others, such as age, smoking, physical activity, and diabetes mellitus, require that we address hypertension and hypercholesterolemia in the overall context of comprehensive patient management.[19]

However, while we may find it difficult, if not impossible, to persuade our patients (or ourselves even) to lose weight and get more exercise (both of which will assist blood pressure control), the development of potent and very successful medications should allow us to control hypertension and hypercholesterolemia in nearly all our patients.

However, the control rates for hypertension show that we are only partially accomplishing our task. In the early days of the national effort to control hypertension, the percentage of adults whose hypertension was controlled was as low as 11%, and this critical rate had improved to only 24% by the 1988–1991 NHANES survey.[20] The most recent comprehensive data from the same survey covers the 1999–2000 period. That survey shows that hypertension control rates have improved to 31%, but *only to 31%*.[21] This undertreatment is not just a US problem, considering that in 2003 hypertension control rates in Canada were only 15.8%.[22]

As we begin to focus on hypertension treatment, there are a number of reasonable questions that might occur to practitioners. These could include: What are the proper criteria for diagnosing hypertension? Are there specific diagnostic techniques beyond office readings that are important? What are our blood pressure targets? In treatment, are there any classes of treatment agents that have been *proven* to have superiority over other treatment choices?

These are important questions, particularly for the busy practitioner, and they will be dealt with at the beginning of this book.

DIAGNOSIS OF HYPERTENSION

Of all the significant health issues we face, the diagnosis of essential hypertension is quite possibly the most important, but certainly the easiest diagnosis that we make. Simply stated, essential hypertension is the presence of blood pressure, properly measured in the office setting, of a systolic pressure of 140 mm Hg or greater, and/or a diastolic pressure of 90 mm Hg or greater (with exceptions as described later). This most routine of procedures, one that can be done easily, inexpensively, with minimal discomfort and no risk to the patient, can identify the prevalence of this most important risk factor for cardiovascular disease.

However, it is important to remember that this diagnosis requires that the pressure be properly measured and repeated at least 1 more session as a repeat visit to make the diagnosis accurately.

OFFICE BLOOD PRESSURE MANAGEMENT

Proper measurement of blood pressure in the office is the cornerstone of hypertension management. There are specific guidelines that, if properly followed, should lead to consistent readings and therefore should properly guide our therapy. Failure to obtain blood pressure readings in a proper manner can lead to underdiagnosis of hypertension (with resultant cardiovascular risk) or overdiagnosis (a much less serious problem) with treatment initiated in a patient who does not yet merit treatment.

The Sixth Report of the Joint National Committee on Prevention, Detection, Evaluation, and Treatment of High Blood Pressure (JNC-VI) identifies the proper technique for office blood pressure measurement.[23]

- Patients should be seated properly, with both feet flat on the floor, with the arm that is to be measured resting on a table at about heart level.
- Patients should be *sitting quietly for at least 5 minutes* before the pressure is measured.
- At the initial visit, both arms should be assessed for cuff size and blood pressure.
- The arm with the *higher* pressure should always be used for measurement.
- At the initial visit, proper cuff size should be determined by measuring the arm circumference. With the patient standing with the arm hanging loosely and the elbow flexed at 90 degrees, measure the length from the proximal humerus to the elbow. Halfway along this length, the diameter of the arm, with the arm still in flexion, should be measured in centimeters.
- For an arm circumference of 24 through 32 centimeters, use a *regular* adult cuff.
- For an arm circumference of 33 through 41 centimeters, use a *large* adult cuff.
- For an arm of greater than 41 centimeters, a small thigh cuff should be used.
- For the *initial diagnosis* of hypertension, blood pressure readings should be repeated at a second visit to confirm the diagnosis. (See Table 1-1.)

Mercury sphygmomanometers are the preferred devices for measurement. If aneroid or electronic devices are utilized, they must be properly and regularly calibrated.

Two or more readings separated by 2 minutes should be averaged to obtain a true reading.

INITIAL EVALUATION[23]

The initial evaluation of a patient with newly diagnosed hypertension should include a medical history, with a focus on cardiovascular risk issues, including diabetes mellitus, hyperlipidemia, and symptomatic coronary, cerebrovascular, or peripheral vascular disease. Family history should include special attention to hypertension and other cardiovascular disease and risk factors. Social history should include smoking history, exercise, diet, alcohol use, and weight patterns.

The physical examination should begin with properly obtained sitting blood pressures, along with a standing blood pressure. The complete examination should emphasize the vascular system, with a careful funduscopic exam, a complete pulmonary exam, a careful cardiac exam, and an examination of the peripheral vascular system, including carotid and abdominal bruits as well as peripheral artery pulses.

Laboratory tests include urinalysis, complete blood count, blood chemistries with a fasting glucose and a fasting lipid panel, along with an electrocardiogram. Other optional tests would be directed by the findings of the examinations and routine testing.

While there is frequently interest in more complicated testing like an echocardiogram, none of the guidelines recommend this expensive test unless there is some clear clinical indication for it.

Table 1-1 Proper Techniques for Measuring Blood Pressure

Initial visit:

Have patient sit quietly with both feet on the floor for 5 minutes.

Measure both arms for proper cuff size, with a regular cuff for arm circumference of 24–32 cm, or a large cuff for 33–41 cm.

Check the pressure in both arms, and do subsequent measurements in the arm with the *higher* readings.

Do at least 2 blood pressure measurements separated by 2 minutes, and use the average of the two.

Follow-up visit:

Have patient sit quietly with both feet on the floor for 5 minutes before taking measurements.

Use proper cuff size, as previously determined.

Use the arm with the higher pressure, as previously determined.

Obtain at least 2 blood pressure readings and average them.

Other techniques for blood pressure measurement are becoming popular, such as home blood pressure measurement and 24-hour ambulatory measurement, but these are optional and are not to take the place of readings obtained by a trained professional in the office environment.

Twenty-Four Hour Ambulatory Measurements

Twenty-four hour ambulatory measurements are regularly used in research, particularly in the trials for new blood pressure medications. The arguments for their more widespread utilization are along the lines that the continuous 24-hour reading renders a more complete record of the pressure. While that position can be argued, there are arguments against regular use of 24-hour monitoring. The most convincing is that there are no clear standards as to what constitutes a normal, borderline, or elevated 24-hour ambulatory blood pressure reading.[24] Indeed, different expert groups in Europe and the United States have different levels of "normal" and "elevated" for 24-hour ambulatory blood pressure readings.[24] Several studies have shown that a subset of patients whose blood pressures do not drop at night ("non-dippers") have a higher rate of cardiovascular events than those patients whose pressure does drop at night ("dippers"). While this is true, it is very difficult to apply in practice, since we do not have any treatment trials based on this type of differentiation of the patients. Until we have treatment trials that can guide us in properly managing medications to treat the "non-dippers" in a different way than we treat traditional hypertensive patients, such as to what level the 24-hour readings should be lowered, the ambulatory 24-hour cuff readings do not offer practical information for use in traditional office practice. Finally, the ambulatory blood pressure cuffs themselves are expensive (and usually not eligible for reimbursement), uncomfortable for the patient to wear, and difficult and time consuming for the staff who administer them. Therefore, I do not encourage their regular use in practice.

Home (or Self) Monitoring

Home (or self) monitoring of blood pressure is also popular with some patients and practitioners. Scientifically, home or self monitoring is limited by the same academic issues that affect 24-hour ambulatory blood pressure monitoring. There is no clear evidence as to what the normal or elevated blood pressure is when monitored by the patient at home.[25] Home blood pressure readings are clearly lower than those obtained in the office, but they are not an accurate substitution for an office-based, professionally measured blood pressure. The risk in encouraging home (self) monitoring is that because home readings are naturally lower than office readings, these home readings might convince the patient that blood pressure treatment is not warranted, when it actually is warranted based upon the office readings. Remember that *all our evidence* of the importance for lowering blood pressure is based on *office* blood pressure readings. I have used home blood pressure monitoring as a safety factor in many blood pressure research trials. I do think it offers a significant psychological benefit for patients and practitioners. If the patient and the practitioner observe the home readings in conjunction with the office readings as therapy evolves, it can serve as an excellent reinforcement to the doctor–patient relationship, which will only improve care.

There is no evidence as to whether the newer, electronic monitors for wrists or fingertip usage offer any value, outside of the potential monitoring during exercise programs. These devises may not be properly calibrated to guarantee accurate readings, so they should be avoided.[26]

White Coat Hypertension

White coat hypertension (the idea that the clinical setting contributes to higher blood pressure levels) is the concern that many patients and practitioners use to justify home or ambulatory measurements. It is controversial whether white coat hypertension truly exists as a distinct entity or is simply the evolution of a patient from normotension through borderline hypertension and into true hypertension. I happen to doubt that white coat hypertension is a real and distinct entity. Physicians and patients need to remember that home blood pressure readings are *naturally* lower outside the office and that *this does not negate the office readings*. Therefore, we must continue to rely on properly done office blood pressure readings to confirm the diagnosis of hypertension.

BLOOD PRESSURE TARGETS

Blood pressure targets have been well studied and confirmed at these current target levels over many years of research. The traditional comprehensive targets of < 140/< 90 mm Hg were confirmed in several studies. The Treatment of Mild Hypertension Study (TOMHS) used a variety of initial therapy agents versus placebo in patients with diastolic blood pressure 90 to 99 mm Hg. Within 1 year, patients on placebo began to demonstrate an increased level of major cardiac events, even at such a mild elevation of pressure.[27] Interestingly, patients on active treatment also had an improved quality of life compared to the patients receiving placebo.[27] That observation would refute the assumption that hypertension is a completely asymptomatic disorder. I have conducted many hypertension research trials that require a washout of therapy followed by a placebo treatment phase. Many patients report a variety of mild symptoms when their pressure is elevated, such as headache, fatigue, and malaise.

The Hypertension Optimal Treatment (HOT) study treated patients to different target levels of diastolic blood pressure (90, 85, or 80 mm Hg, respectively) to determine if there was a level of treated blood pressure "too low," also known as the "J-curve" phenomenon.[28] The HOT study did *not* show any evidence for a "too low," or "J-curve," effect since there was not an increase in cardiovascular events in the patients with noticeably lower blood pressures.[29] The lowest level of cardiac events were in patients treated to the 132–136/82–86 mm Hg range, confirming the traditional targets of < 140/< 90 mm Hg for general hypertension patients. Stroke was the only endpoint that continued to decline slightly in incidence as the blood pressure was lowered further. However, the HOT study did show that more aggressive treatment and lower pressures did produce benefit in diabetic patients.[29]

BLOOD PRESSURE TARGETS IN COMPLICATED PATIENTS

While the traditional blood pressure targets of < 140/90 mm Hg are sufficient for uncomplicated patients, there are 4 patient subgroups where the targets have been lowered to the level of < 130/80 mm Hg. Four conditions have been identified for the < 130/80 mm Hg targets: diabetes mellitus, chronic kidney disease, ischemic heart disease, and heart failure.[30–32] (See Table 1-2.)

In Table 2, the lower target levels for diabetes are derived from the benefit from lower target levels seen in the HOT study and from consensus guidelines. The lower targets for chronic kidney are for patients with reduced renal function, defined as a serum creatinine of > 1.5 mg/dL in men and > 1.3 mg/dL in women, or albuminuria of > 300 mg/day.[30] The lower targets for patients with ischemic heart disease are from a recent American Heart

Table 1-2 Target Blood Pressures

Uncomplicated patients:

< 140/90 mm Hg

Complicated patients with hypertension and:

Diabetes Mellitus: < 130/80 mm Hg

Chronic kidney disease or proteinuria: < 130/80 mm Hg

Ischemic heart disease: < 130/80 mm Hg

Heart failure: < 130/80 mm Hg

Association Scientific Statement, and the Heart Failure guidelines are from a Heart Failure Society of America consensus statement.

These lowered targets can present an increased challenge for practitioners. Many of the patients with the complicating conditions are on multiple medications for their complicated problems already, and achieving these targets may appear daunting. Also, the number of adult Americans with 1 or more of these conditions will be in the tens of millions, illustrating the enormous task ahead for practitioners to meet these targets.

Chapter 2
Hypertension Management

The most challenging question surrounding hypertension management is whether there is a specific class (or classes) of agent that provides superior protection against cardiovascular events compared to other classes of agents. The argument began with the JNC-IV report issued in 1988, which sited a "preference" for initiating hypertension therapy with diuretics and beta-blockers. They based their preference on the fact that only those 2 classes, principally diuretics, had been proven to reduce cardiovascular events (primarily stroke). However, this recommendation was not supported by specific trials that had used beta-blockers as initial therapy, like the trials where diuretics had been used. Nonetheless, beta-blockers were recommended, even though specific clinical trial evidence to support this recommendation was lacking. Since diuretics and beta-blockers were the only antihypertensive agent classes that were generic at the time of that report, many of us thought the primary motivation behind the recommendation was financial, in an effort to lower medication expenses.

Recently, the issues have evolved quite a bit. In general, many classes of antihypertensive agents, including the ACE inhibitors, calcium channel blockers (CCBs), alpha-blockers, and longer acting beta-blockers have had their patents expire and have been supplanted by low-cost generic versions. For practitioners and patients, this means we have the option of a wide variety of inexpensive medications to control hypertension.

Scientifically, a series of trials has examined the question as to whether one class or combination of classes is superior in reducing cardiac events. The most well known of these efforts was a very large US trial called ALLHAT. ALLHAT compared a diuretic, chlorthalidone, to a CCB (amlodipine), and to an ACE inhibitor (lisinopril).[33] There was no difference in the rate of overall cardiac events between the groups, showing equal efficacy between the agents. While supporters of diuretic superiority claim that differences in secondary endpoints like heart failure show superiority for chlorthalidone, this claim is not true. In any equivalence study, even if the primary endpoint is equivalent, there will frequently be some difference in secondary endpoints. However, the overall equivalence of the primary endpoint firmly supports equivalency. If the primary endpoint is equivalent, then the treatments are equivalent. Therefore, ALLHAT does not support superiority for diuretics.

Several trials directly compared various CCBs with diuretics or beta-blockers, or both, and they all showed equivalency in reducing overall cardiovascular events.[34–36] One atherosclerosis trial compared a CCB to atenolol with no difference in cardiovascular events.[37] One trial, VALUE, compared amlodipine, a calcium channel inhibitor, to valsartan, an angiotensin II inhibitor, and, after correction for different levels of blood pressure control, found equivalent cardiovascular events.[38,39]

Interestingly, there are 2 studies that directly challenge the diuretic-first hypothesis. ASCOT-BPLA was a large hypertension treatment comparison trial in northwest Europe.[40] It measured fatal and nonfatal MI rates in a regimen of the beta-blocker atenolol and a thiazide diuretic versus a regimen of amlodipine, a CCB, and an ACE inhibitor, perindopril. The primary endpoint showed a strong, but not quite significant reduction in events in the latter group, with a significant reduction in a variety of powerful endpoints like overall mortality and cardiovascular events and procedures. This study documents that the traditional atenolol/thiazide regimen was not superior to a CCB/ACE inhibitor regimen. A similar pattern of a marginal, but clear superiority of an ACE inhibitor-based regimen over a diuretic-based regimen, particularly in men, was seen in a study of elderly hypertension patients in Australia.[41] A recently reported trial, ACCOMPLISH, compared a regimen combining benazapril (ACE inhibitor) with amlodipine (a CCB) versus benazapril combined with HCTZ (hydrochlorothiazide, a diuretic) in doses of 12.5 to 25 mg. The benazapril/amlodipine group had a 20% reduction in cardiovascular morbidity and mortality compared to the benazapril/HCTZ group, a dramatic result that was powerful and clear and challenges the diuretic preference hypothesis.[42]

As in most of medicine, these studies are somewhat conflicting and confusing, particularly for the busy practitioner. In summary, I think the overall message from these studies is that it's not *how* you control the pressure, but *that* you control the pressure that is important. I think each practitioner should feel free to choose the right agent or combination of agents best suited for each individual patient. In this context, you should feel free to consider many factors, such as the patient's comorbid conditions, potential for side effects, cost, ease of dosing, age, and systolic and diastolic values. Remember to focus on controlling the blood pressure in a way that is successful and accommodating to the needs of the patient.

COMPELLING INDICATIONS

The JNC-VII identifies a number of "Compelling Indications" where certain classes of antihypertensive agents should be used. These indications are derived from a large number of clinical trials. Some of these trials were designed to evaluate the particular effectiveness of the agents in reducing cardiovascular events in specific situations, such as beta-blockers in patients with a recent MI, and some are drawn from consensus guidelines from expert panels. In many situations, the use of these agents will not only lower the blood pressure, but it will also protect against further cardiovascular or other serious events. In a number of patients—for instance, patients with recent acute coronary syndrome or heart failure—we will be compelled to use multiple agents that will not only treat hypertension but will also prevent further cardiovascular or renal conditions. The accepted compelling indications are listed in the following paragraphs, and in Table 2-1.

Table 2-1 Compelling Indications for Concurrent Medical Conditions

High-Risk Conditions with Compelling Indications	Recommended Drugs					
	Diuretic	Beta-Blocker	ACE-I	ARB	CCB	Aldosterone Antagonist
Heart Failure	x	x	x	x		x
Post-MI		x	x			x
High CHD Risk	x	x	x		x	
Diabetes	x	x	x	x	x	
Chronic Kidney Disease			x	x		
Recurrent CVA Prevention	x		x			

The background behind the use of each agent for specific indications will be discussed in the individual treatment chapters. The indications need to be observed carefully, since in many situations, only certain agents in each class, and at certain doses, have actually been studied properly to confirm their effectiveness. The best example is the use of beta-blockers in heart failure. Three beta-blocker preparations have been proven effective in reducing cardiac events or mortality in patients with heart failure: extended release metoprolol (Toprol XL) in doses of 100 to 200 mg, carvedilol (Coreg) in doses titrated to 25 mg twice daily, and bisoprolol at 10 mg daily.[43–45] However, a different beta-blocker, bucindolol, which is not on the US market, *did not* reduce cardiac events in a similar study in heart failure patients.[46] Finally, in the COMET trial, full-dose carvedilol, when compared to low doses of 50 mg twice daily of immediate-release metoprolol, was found to be superior in reducing cardiac events in heart failure patients.[47] Looking at these studies in detail emphasizes the importance of carefully considering the available scientific data as we make our decisions. As such, in the US, we should use only extended release metoprolol (Toprol XL) or carvedilol (Coreg) in the doses used in their successful studies to treat heart failure patients. Even though atenolol is a widely used beta-blocker, it has not been studied in heart failure, so we do not know what dose and dose schedule might be effective, if any.

The compelling indications, as defined by the JNC-VII recommendations, are as follows:

Heart failure: diuretics, beta-blockers (certain agents), ACE inhibitors, angiotensin receptor blockers (ARBs), aldosterone antagonist

Post-MI: beta-blockers, ACE inhibitors, aldosterone antagonist

High coronary risk: diuretics, beta-blockers, ACE inhibitors, CCBs (and probably ARBs in the future)

Diabetes: diuretics, beta-blockers, ACE inhibitors, ARBs, CCBs

Chronic kidney disease: ACE inhibitors, ARBs

Recurrent stroke prevention: diuretics, ACE inhibitors

MULTIPLE AGENT THERAPY

One of the most compelling questions for practitioners in the management of hypertension revolves around the use of multiple medications. Many of us are accustomed to using 2 combinations, say an ACE inhibitor with a diuretic, to treat blood pressure, but is it acceptable to use 3, 4, or more hypertensive medications? What about side effects, or the cost of the medications?

These are all legitimate concerns, but they need to be evaluated in the context of the risk of uncontrolled hypertension. The side effects of uncontrolled or poorly controlled hypertension are severe, including stroke, heart attack, heart failure, and early death or disability. Also, the *cost* of these cardiovascular events, both to the patients and the healthcare system are immense and are much greater than the cost of multiple medications. Therefore, we need to adjust our thinking so that *control* of the blood pressure is the goal. Many of the side effects we worry about, such as pedal edema from CCBs, are cosmetic only and otherwise are inconsequential.

Evidence supports the use of multiple medications. A Veterans Affairs (VA) study in the 1990s showed that in men with diastolic blood pressure between 95 mm Hg and 109 mm Hg, *antihypertensive monotherapy* reduced the diastolic pressure to < 90 mm Hg only about 50% of the time.[48] Indeed, in research protocols where the investigator is compelled to increase medications to reach target blood pressures, many patients were titrated to *3 or more medications* to achieve the goal.[49]

Indeed, the JNC-VII report recommends considering initiating therapy with a 2-drug combination, like an ACE inhibitor/thiazide combination, if the untreated pressures are > 20/10 mm Hg above the target pressures.[30] In general, outside of the unusual situation where the pressures are critically high, like > 180 mm Hg systolic or > 110 mm Hg diastolic, gradual titration of medications is indicated. In noncritical situations, patients should be seen at least monthly while titrating medication for elevated pressure.[30] This follow-up reveals the full effect of the new medication or increased dose.

INITIATING HYPERTENSION THERAPY

Deciding how to initiate therapy (or even to titrate existing therapy) is where our knowledge of the treatment agents mixes with our understanding of the patient. We should ask ourselves a series of questions as we begin to make these decisions.

These questions include:

Is the pressure so elevated (> 20/10 mm Hg above targets) that we should consider dual or combination therapy as initial therapy?

What is the type of elevated pressure we are going to treat: mixed systolic/diastolic elevation, isolated systolic elevation, or diastolic hypertension?

Does the patient have any compelling conditions such as diabetes that will direct our therapy?

What is the patient's age? What is the patient's ethnicity? Is the patient a fertile female?

Does the patient have preferences regarding the type of therapy, such as the least expensive treatment or the treatment with the lowest risk of side effects?

How important is it to me that my choice of initial therapy has been specifically proven to reduce cardiovascular events in this type of patient when used as initial therapy?

Potential answers should help us decide on how to initiate therapy.

In situations of significant elevations of > 20/10 mm Hg above the target, it is reasonable and common to initiate therapy with a combination product, like a combination of a thiazide diuretic with an ACE inhibitor, ARB, or beta-blocker.

There are many other combinations or potential combinations available. One consideration of initiating therapy with a fixed combination product is that you will have to have the patient switch to a new product if you feel the need to increase one of the components of the combination at a subsequent visit. Therefore, it might be prudent initially to give the agents separately and then to go to a combination product when the pressure is controlled and the doses of both agents are stable.

Different types of elevated pressures sometimes point us toward specific therapies. Isolated systolic pressure, seen almost exclusively in the elderly, responds very well to thiazide diuretic therapy, usually initiated at 12.5 mg of hydrochlorothiazide or chlorthalidone. Also, ACE inhibitors and dihydropyridine CCBs have been proven safe and effective in this type of patient. In patients with mixed systolic/diastolic hypertension or predominantly diastolic hypertension, many of the traditional classes of agents are acceptable and effective. ACE inhibitors are excellent choices, along with CCBs (particularly the dihydropyridines like amlodipine or felodopine) and of course the diuretics. The ASCOT study result has led some physicians to question the role of beta-blockers as initial therapy in patients such as these, unless there is a compelling indication (preferring to use them as add-on medication in more complicated patients). Any of these agents could be started at either their initial or moderate therapeutic doses, depending on the patient.

Compelling indications are very important, and they are detailed previously. In many situations, like the presence of recent or even remote acute coronary syndrome, the use (per guidelines) of beta-blockers and ACE inhibitors (or ARBs instead) may control the pressure even to the lower targets of < 130/80 mm Hg. If not, other therapy should be added in an appropriate time frame. Similar issues are important in the heart failure patient or the diabetic patient. If a patient has glucose intolerance or even metabolic syndrome, initiating ACE inhibitor or ARB therapy may slow the development of diabetes and avoid the necessity of adding one of those agents when diabetes does develop.

Older patients tend to have noticeably fewer side effects from diuretic therapy than we frequently see from younger patients. Since they predominantly have systolic elevations, diuretics are often very useful in older patients. African American patients respond somewhat differently than white patients. This difference, with a potent response to thiazide diuretics and CCBs, is less than many practitioners suppose. There is a misconception that African Americans do not respond well to ACE inhibitors or ARBs. However, a careful look at the research data shows that the response of African American patients is nearly the

Table 2-2 Considerations for Initial Therapy

Agent	Patient Characteristics
ACE-Inhibitors	All patients appropriate except fertile or pregnant females Crucial in patients with CHD, HF, AODM, renal disease
Beta-Blockers	Doubts about use as initial therapy Crucial in patients with CHD or HF
Calcium Channel Blockers	All patients appropriate Useful in African Americans and elderly with systolic hypertension Useful in CHD and AODM
Diuretics	All patients appropriate Special efficacy in elderly with systolic hypertension and in African Americans, and in patients with HF or previous CVA
Angiotensin Receptor Blockers	All patients appropriate except fertile or pregnant females Special efficacy in AODM, renal disease, and CHD

same as white patients, but that African American patients require the maximum doses to be effective.

Patient satisfaction with their own hypertension therapy is critical, and their preferences should be understood. For patients, often younger and very busy, where avoidance of side effects is paramount, ARBs are generally free of side effects. ACE inhibitors are usually free of side effects, with the exception of cough, and CCB side effects (edema, flushing, and constipation) are usually mild and self-limited. If affordability is the priority, diuretics are very useful. Also, many of the ACE inhibitors and CCBs are now generic and much less expensive. Even long-acting beta-blockers like extended release metoprolol are now generic, and the ARBs are in the process of becoming generic. Therefore, managing hypertension in an affordable way is not difficult.

As I have stated earlier, I do not hold to the belief that diuretics have been proven to be superior to other classes of agents and therefore must be used as initial therapy. While there are clearly some patients who will benefit from diuretic therapy, like elderly patients with isolated systolic pressure, there is clear evidence that other therapeutic classes, specifically ACE inhibitors and CCBs, are equally effective in reducing cardiovascular events. Only beta-blockers, based on ASCOT, have been questioned recently as initial therapy. ARBs have not been studied as initial therapy in uncomplicated hypertension, but their success in reducing events in complicated patients supports considering them as appropriate first-line therapy also. (See Table 2-2.)

Chapter 3

Diuretics

Diuretics come in 4 distinctive molecular groups, generally with different pharmacological properties and uses. The one exception is the similarity between the thiazides and indapamide, an indole derivative. Indapamide is structurally distinct from the thiazides, but its effects, and therefore its utilization, are very similar to the thiazides. The thiazides have excellent effectiveness in reducing blood pressure, but they have very limited effect in reducing edema from heart or renal failure. Therefore, the thiazides need to be regarded as a treatment for high blood pressure rather than for volume overload.

The loop diuretics (furosemide and others) are extremely potent in stimulating the excretion of sodium and fluid volume, but they have limited blood pressure lowering effects in the absence of significant volume overload. Therefore, the use of the loop diuretics should be confined to volume overload situations like heart or renal failure. The potassium-sparing diuretics are a different class of agents that work farther down the renal tubular system in the distal tubule and retain potassium in exchange for sodium. They are rarely used alone, since they are weak diuretics. They are frequently used in combination with thiazide diuretic preparations. One agent, spironolactone, has been shown to be useful in severe heart failure, along with its traditional use in primary hyperaldosteronism.

THIAZIDE DIURETICS

Thiazide diuretics have been and will remain a fundamental treatment modality in the management of hypertension. Long associated with the treatment of hypertension, they remain integral to our management of the disease.

Thiazides have been comprehensively studied in a wide variety of types of hypertension, and they remain a fundamental class of agents across the spectrum of the disease. The original "moderate" (now stage I-II hypertension) trial used chlorthalidone as the original treatment.[11] Many other studies have used either chlorthalidone, hydrochlorothiazide (HCTZ), or other similar agents used in other parts of the world.

Mechanism of Action

The mechanism of action of the antihypertensive effect for the thiazide diuretics is unclear, but it does *not* appear to be directly related to the diuretic effect.[50] With the onset of thiazide therapy, there is a modest diuresis that reduces both intracellular and extracellular fluid. This diuresis is modest and quickly stabilizes. It can result in a temporary reduction in cardiac output, but this, along with the drop in intravascular volume, is only transient. This diuresis does lead to an activation of the renin-angiotensin-aldosterone system (RAAS), which can have some enhancement of blood pressure. However, these diuretic effects are relatively transient, and the activation of the RAAS has limited effect on the rate of blood pressure reduction. The thiazides lower blood pressure by reducing arterial vascular resistance through a mechanism(s) that is unclear even after 40 years of use.

The characteristics of the commonly used thiazide diuretics and their traditional doses are listed in Table 3-1.

Evidence of Efficacy

Thiazide diuretics were the original therapeutic agents active from the beginning of the war against hypertension. As noted earlier, the original VA trial in 1967 used HCTZ (along with reserpine and hydralazine) against placebo, with significant reduction in stroke and heart failure.[10] The follow-up VA study published in 1970 also compared HCTZ, again along with reserpine and hydralazine, to placebo in patients with diastolic blood pressure from 90 to 114 mm Hg.[11] This study also showed a reduction in stroke and heart failure. The Australian

Table 3-1 Thiazide Diuretics

	Dosage/day	Half-life (hrs)	Duration Action (hrs)
Chlorthalidone	12.5–50 mg	35–50	24–72
Hydrochlorothiazide	12.5–50 mg	6–15	12–18
Methyclothiazide	2.5–5 mg		> 24
Metolazone	0.5–5 mg	14	18–24

study treated mild hypertension with chlorothiazide, with other second- and third-level drugs added if necessary.[51] Cardiovascular events were significantly reduced by the active treatment. The MRC trial in the United Kingdom, also in mild hypertension, used bendrofluzide or propranolol versus placebo.[52] This study also showed a reduction in stroke but not in heart attack. All of the previously mentioned trials were in middle-aged patients.

Several trials with mixed systolic and diastolic hypertension were undertaken. The STOP-2 trial was a Swedish trial in the elderly, comparing HCTZ/amiloride, metoprolol, atenolol, or pindolol against placebo, with significant reductions in cardiovascular and stroke deaths in the treatment groups.[53] The MRC Elderly trial also used HCTZ/amiloride, atenolol, or placebo.[54] The diuretic-treated group had reductions in stroke, coronary events, and cardiovascular events compared to placebo.

In patients with isolated systolic hypertension in the SHEP study (Systolic Hypertension in the Elderly), the elderly patients were randomized to chlorthalidone or placebo.[14] The patients on thiazide had reduced stroke, fatal and nonfatal MI, and cardiovascular events.

In an overview of these trials, thiazide diuretics showed particular potency to reduce stroke and heart failure, along with MI in the elderly, when used to treat all types of hypertension.

Agents and Dosage

The current doses of thiazide diuretics commonly used are significantly lower than the doses used in the past. In general, 12.5 mg of HCTZ or chlorthalidone is used as initial therapy, rather than the 50 mg doses used in decades past. The use of these much lower doses has allowed for a significant reduction in the number and severity of the side effects, which become quite prominent as the dose increases, particularly to the 50 mg dose. The 12.5 mg doses of HCTZ or chlorthalidone are generally well tolerated and reduce the risk of long-term side effects, particularly hypokalemia. The 12.5 mg dose has therefore become the traditional dose when a thiazide is added as a supplementary agent to existing therapy.

Initial doses of HCTZ or chlorthalidone depend on the patient's situation. In the SHEP study of elderly patients being treated for isolated systolic hypertension, the initial dose was 12.5 mg of chlorthalidone, with titration to 25 mg, if necessary. In this group of patients with systolic elevation only, the 12.5 mg initial dose controlled the systolic blood pressure in only 30% of patients, with an additional 16% being controlled when the dose was titrated up to 25 mg.[14] In general, this study highlights that much of the thiazide blood pressure reduction is seen at the initial 12.5 mg dose, with only a modest increase in control rates with the doubled dose. This type of relatively flat dose response curve is typical for many agents. Therefore, in routine situations, initiating thiazide diuretics at the 12.5 mg dose is reasonable.

Adding a thiazide diuretic to a patient already taking 1 or more antihypertensives follows a similar pattern. It is quite common, even typical, to add a small dose of thiazide to a patient who is not completely controlled on an ACE inhibitor or ARB. Frequently these are patients where the initial therapy has controlled the diastolic pressure but has not completely controlled the systolic pressure. Since the ACE inhibitor or ARB has already inhibited the RAAS, this will avoid activation of the RAAS by the thiazide, resulting in a synergistic effect between the 2 therapies. This type of combination has been very popular, and that led to most manufacturers producing ACE inhibitor or ARB products combined with 12.5 mg of HCTZ. In many situations, however, the initial dose of 12.5 mg of thiazide may not be enough to control the systolic hypertension, and an increase to 25 mg is necessary. This treatment has become increasingly important in the last 5 years, as difficult-to-control systolic blood pressure has become more of a priority here in the United States. Manufacturers have responded recently, with many ACE inhibitor or ARB combination pills now having the option of either a 12.5 or 25 mg dose of HCTZ. The advantages and difficulties of this regimen are illustrated by the MATRIX study of irbesartan and HCTZ combinations. The 25 mg HCTZ dose produced a significant 6 to 7 mm Hg reduction in the systolic blood pressure over the 12.5 mg dose, an important therapeutic success.[55] However, the 25 mg HCTZ did produce greater reductions in serum potassium than did the 12.5 mg dose, even though this was somewhat ameliorated when the patients were on therapeutic doses of the ARB irbesartan.[55]

Thiazide diuretics can also be added to therapy as third or even later-step agents, if the patient's situation indicates it. The dosing process should follow the same pattern of 12.5 mg as initial therapy in most patients. We should note that the JNC-VI expects that a 3-drug regimen should include a diuretic.[23]

Side Effects

Side effects remain a considerable issue with the use of thiazide diuretics. The rate of side effects is difficult to determine clearly, so our opinions, and those of our patients, are shaped by our experience. Determining the actual rate of side effects is difficult and often somewhat controversial. This difficulty is increased because many of the early diuretic studies did not evaluate the rate of side effects, understandably concentrating on the rates of cardiovascular events.

There is consensus on one factor, that the side effects of diuretics are dose dependent, and therefore using the lowest effective dose will lessen the side effect impact. I will categorize the effects in 3 categories: electrolyte problems, generalized somatic complaints, and metabolic abnormalities.

Electrolyte Problems

Electrolyte problems are the most obvious side effects seen with thiazides. Hypokalemia is the most serious, but also best-understood consequence of long-term diuretic therapy. It has been reported in nearly all long-term diuretic trials.[14,27,33,56] While hypokalemia can lead to serious ventricular arrhythmias, the absolute risk of this is unclear.[57] However, the potential for this problem remains and mandates that we monitor for potassium depletion and treat it when detected. Hyponatremia can also occur, but with less frequency than hyperkalemia. Hyponatremia usually requires simply the discontinuation of the diuretic, while hypokalemia can be managed by a wide variety of potassium replacement products. Many practitioners have used combinations of diuretics with triamterene or amiloride, agents that have mild potassium-retaining properties, in an effort to avoid hypokalemia.

Generalized Somatic Complaints

Generalized somatic complaints include fatigue, impotence, lightheadedness, and other often vague symptoms. These types of symptoms were not detected in the TOMHS study, which compared multiple antihypertensive agents to placebo.[27] The NORDIL study, which compared diuretic-based treatment with treatment based on the CCB diltiazem, found significantly higher rates of fatigue and impotence in the diuretic group.[34] These symptoms are often quite important to the affected patients, so we must be sensitive to them and inquire if they are occurring during diuretic therapy.

Metabolic Abnormalities

Metabolic abnormalities include an increase in glucose intolerance and an increase in lipid fraction pathology. Whether the effects showing an increase in cholesterol fade over the years or persist is controversial, with conflicting data from the few studies that have studied this.[58,59] However, any increase in lipid abnormalities can be easily managed by lipid therapy. Persistent elevations in blood glucose are much more ominous, as we face an epidemic of type II diabetes mellitus. A number of studies have shown the elevation of blood glucose, even to the point of frank diabetes, is linked to thiazide therapy.[14,33,59] The high rate of metabolic syndrome and diabetes among hypertensive patients needs to be remembered as we contemplate which agents to use to control blood pressure.

Thiazides also produce increased urinary retention of uric acid and calcium. The hyperuricemia can present a problem in patients with gout. The calcium retention has meant the thiazides have become a treatment to prevent recurrent calcium-based kidney stones.

OTHER DIURETICS

Indapamide

Indapamide (Lozol) is an indoline diuretic that has a different molecular structure from the thiazides. It has diuretic and hypotensive effects similar to the thiazides, with minimal metabolic effects at the lower doses of 1.25 mg and 2.5 mg. Recently it has been marketed in combination with the ACE inhibitor perindopril with an indication to reduce recurrent stroke.

Metolazone

Metolazone is a diuretic that works at the proximal tubule, a site of action different than any other agent. It is not widely used in routine hypertension. It is sometimes used for diuresis in renal failure patients where diuresis is unsuccessful with loop diuretics alone. Great caution to avoid excess diuresis is important when combining potent diuretics that act at different areas in the tubules and loops, because the potential for significant electrolyte abnormalities from the diuresis is quite high.

Loop Diuretics

The loop diuretics include furosemide, bumetadine, torsemide, and ethacrynic acid. These agents all work in the nephron by blocking sodium reabsorption in the loop of Henle. These agents produce a potent diuresis with significant excretion of fluid, sodium, and potassium. Because of their relatively short half-life and limited hypotensive effects, in general, these agents are *not* used to control blood pressure in uncomplicated hypertension.

In patients who are retaining significant excess volume from heart and/or renal failure, these agents have considerable value. Indeed, patients with difficult-to-control hypertension who have excess volume on board from heart and/or renal failure may need treatment with a loop diuretic, at least temporarily, to reduce the excess volume before the blood pressure can be controlled. This is a limited use where loop diuretics are crucial, but this does not lead to their regular use in the management of hypertension.

Potassium-Sparing Diuretics

There are 3 potassium-sparing diuretics: amiloride, triamterene, and spironolactone. Spironolactone has enjoyed a resurgence in use recently as a late agent in severe heart failure. Because of the severity of the disease and the use of multiple other medications, this use requires great caution and close monitoring of renal function and potassium and other electrolytes.

In the past, these 3 agents, which produce a modest diuresis, were combined with HCTZ as combination products to reduce the risk of hypokalemia from the thiazide. Recently, there has been attention paid to the detection of elevated aldosterone as a cause of difficult-to-control hypertension along with unexplained hypokalemia. Spironolactone is the treatment of choice for elevated aldosterone. The potassium and renal function should be monitored, and breast enlargement can be a common symptomatic side effect in men.

Chapter 4

Angiotensin-Converting Enzyme Inhibitors—ACE Inhibitors

Angiotensin-converting enzyme inhibitors, or ACE inhibitors, are premier agents in the management of hypertension and many other aspects of cardiovascular disease. They offer the practitioner an outstanding pattern of excellent potency in controlling blood pressure, additional benefits in protecting patients with other cardiovascular and metabolic problems, and a low level of side effects. In most situations, an ACE inhibitor is my initial patient choice because of its efficacy and excellent tolerance, and this is supported by the recommendation of the JNC-VII.[30] By initiating ACE inhibitor therapy at the beginning, the patients will already be on this very protective therapy if they are to develop one of the many cardiovascular or metabolic problems—coronary artery disease, heart failure, renal failure, or diabetes—that are common in hypertensive patients.

Finally, many, and soon all, of these valuable agents have become generic, making them very affordable. The generic medications include many of the once-daily preparations, which makes dosing, and hopefully patient acceptance, much easier.

MECHANISM OF ACTION

The mechanism of action of the ACE inhibitor agents is complex and briefly outlined in Figure 4-1. However, within a few months after the initiation of ACE inhibitor therapy, the angiotensin II levels have routinely returned to normal, through accessory pathways of production. Recent information has demonstrated that the renin-angiotensin system is

Renin Angiotensin System

Angiotensinogen

Renin → → ↓ Renin Inhibitors block here

Angiotensin I

ACE → → ↓ ACE Inhibitors block here

Angiotensin II

← ← ↓ → →

↓ ↓

AT I receptor AT II receptor

Vasoconstriction → → ↑**BP**↑ ← ←↑ Aldosterone secretion

Angiotensin Receptors (ARBs) Block
at the AT I receptor

Figure 4-1 Mechanism of Action for ACE Inhibitors

also located intracellularly in many tissues, further complicating our understanding of the mechanisms.

While it was initially assumed that the major mechanism of ACE inhibitors was directly due to the reduction of systemic angiotensin II production, that mechanism now appears to be of limited importance, with other mechanisms, particularly moderation of the bradykinin system, being more important. In the bradykinin system, the angiotensin-converting enzyme is crucial in the transformation of bradykinin into inactive peptides. This breakdown is moderated by the angiotensin-converting enzyme. Blocking this enzyme with an ACE inhibitor thus leads to an accumulation of bradykinin, which is a potent vasodilator compound. However, this accumulation of bradykinin also appears to lead to some of the most significant side effects of the ACE inhibitors, namely angioedema and cough.

EVIDENCE OF EFFICACY

ACE inhibitors are one of the most completely studied and valuable classes of cardiovascular agents ever developed. Initially developed for severe hypertension, they were rapidly understood to treat all stages of hypertension very well, with an acceptable level of side effects. In a series of landmark trials from the early 1990s through the present, aggressive ACE inhibitor therapy has been shown to reduce cardiovascular events in a very wide array of patients. Several different ACE inhibitor agents were shown to reduce total and cardiac mortality, heart failure, MI, and hospitalization in patients with heart failure or left ventricular dysfunction after infarction.[60–63] In the EUROPA study, perindopril reduced cardiovascular events in stable patients with previous MI but with a normal ejection fraction.[64] In the pivotal HOPE study, ramipril reduced mortality and a wide range of other cardiovascular events in patients with previous vascular events or diabetes but with a normal ejection fraction.[65] In the PROGRESS study, a combination treatment of perindopril and the diuretic indapamide reduced recurrent stroke and cardiovascular events in patients with previous cerebrovascular disease.[66]

The agents have also been shown to slow the progression of renal decline in diabetic and other renal failure patients, and to protect against the development of early coronary heart disease that is seen frequently in diabetic patients.[67–70] In the HOPE study, the patients who received ramipril had a significantly lower rate of the development of *new* diabetes, suggesting a positive effect on glucose metabolism.[65] A similar benefit was suggested in a similar trial, where ramipril reduced the level of glucose intolerance but not frank diabetes.[71]

Finally, in patients with left ventricular hypertrophy, ACE inhibitors were more potent than diuretics and beta-blockers at reducing the left ventricular mass index.[72]

AGENTS AND DOSAGE

There are currently 10 ACE inhibitors available on the US market, with others available in other nations. Most of the newer agents, with the exception of the original agents of captopril and enalapril (which must be dosed twice daily) are effective in once-daily doses. Details for the agents are in Table 4-1. In patients with heart failure, half-strength initial doses are recommended for the initial doses with some agents, particularly captopril, enalapril, lisinopril, quinapril, and trandolapril, with subsequent titration to the full doses. Please note that all of the long-term trials mentioned previously titrated the ACE inhibitors to the maximum dose, so those doses should be used in treatment of the cardiovascular, renal, and diabetic protection situations discussed.

Table 4-1 ACE Inhibitors

Agent	Doses	Dosing Schedule
Benazepril (*Lotensin*)	5–40 mg	Once daily
Captopril (*Capoten*)	12.5–50 mg	Two to three times daily
Enalapril (*Vasotec*)	10–40 mg	Once or twice daily
Fosinopril (*Monopril*)	10–40 mg	Once daily
Lisinopril (*Prinivil/Zestril*)	10–40 mg	Once daily
Moexipril (*Univasc*)	7.5–15 mg	Once or twice daily
Perindopril (*Aceon*)	4–8 mg	Once daily
Quinapril (*Accupril*)	10–40 mg	Once or twice daily

Table 4-1 ACE Inhibitors (cont'd)

Agent	Doses	Dosing Schedule
Ramipril (*Altace*)	2.5–10 mg	Once daily
Trandolapril (*Mavik*)	1–4 mg	Once daily

In cases of significant renal failure, usually with a creatinine clearance of < 30 mL/min, doses should be reduced to half the usual dose. Fosinopril, which is cleared both renally and hepatically, does not have to make this adjustment.

Caution: Any of the ACE inhibitors can lead to fetal injury if given to pregnant females. Since many pregnancies are unplanned, I recommend against using ACE inhibitors (or ARBs) in fertile females at any time. If you think the use of an ACE inhibitor or ARB is essential for a fertile female, great caution should be taken regarding contraception, and a consultation(s) would probably be appropriate before starting therapy.

SIDE EFFECTS

Cough

The side effect pattern of the ACE inhibitors is generally mild and well tolerated. Cough is the most common side effect. The cough is dry without sputum or dyspnea. It is caused by a "dry, tickle in the throat" sensation, and some patients feel it is worse at night. It can easily be confused with the irritation of allergic rhinitis or postnasal drip, but there is no rhinorrhea with ACE inhibitor cough. The cough will cease very quickly with the cessation of the ACE inhibitor, and this is the real diagnostic test. The cough can be caused by any of the ACE inhibitors, but the *rate of cough* varies between the agents. In the only head-to-head trial, fosinopril had about half the rate of cough as did enalapril.[73] As you use these agents, pay attention to the rate of cough seen with various agents, and adjust your prescribing accordingly. If a patient has a critical indication for an ACE inhibitor but cannot take one due to severe cough, switching to one of the more potent of the ARBs, like telmisartan, candasartan, or irbesartan, may be appropriate.

Angioedema

Angioedema is the most serious side effect of ACE inhibitors. It can present as a relatively mild swelling of the lips or face, or it can rapidly become a life-threatening swelling of the upper airway. It is, fortunately, a very rare complication, but when it appears in a patient taking an ACE inhibitor, the drug must be stopped immediately and not resumed. Referral of the patient to the emergency department for airway management is often necessary.

Other Side Effects

Other side effects have been reported with the ACE inhibitors, including hyperkalemia, which will rarely become significant, but requires monitoring. Very careful monitoring for hyperkalemia is important when an ACE inhibitor is combined with other agents that can also lead to potassium retention. This is particularly important when an ACE inhibitor is combined with an ARB for hypertension or heart failure management, and especially with spironolactone in heart failure patients. Renal decline has been seen with ACE inhibitor therapy, but this is rare and often related to bilateral renal artery stenosis or renal artery stenosis in a solitary kidney, which are quite rare. Alterations in white blood counts have also been reported, but this is also rare.

COMBINATION THERAPY

Six of the ACE inhibitors on the US market have combination preparations, all of which involve combinations of ACE inhibitor with various doses of HCTZ. The combination of these agent classes is very sound pharmacologically, with the ACE inhibitor providing inhibition of the renin-angiotensin system, which often is enhanced by the effect of the HCTZ. Therefore, this combination of agents is usually very effective.

The available combination products and their various doses are listed in Table 4-2.

Table 4-2 Combination ACE/HCTZ Preparations

ACE-Inhibitor	ACE Dose	HCTZ Dose
Benazepril (*Lotensin HCT*)	5 mg 10 mg 20 mg 20 mg	6.25 mg 12.5 mg 12.5 mg 25 mg
Captopril (*Capozide*)	25 mg 25 mg 50 mg 50 mg	15 mg 25 mg 15 mg 25 mg
Enalapril (*Vaseretic*)	5 mg 10 mg	12.5 mg 25 mg
Lisinopril (*Prinzide, Zestoretic*)	10 mg 20 mg 20 mg	12.5 mg 12.5 mg 25 mg
Moexipril (*Uniretic*)	7.5 mg 15 mg	12.5 mg 25 mg
Quinapril (*Accuretic*)	10 mg 20 mg 20 mg	12.5 mg 12.5 mg 25 mg

Whether and how to use these fixed-dose preparations is a highly individual decision. When the ACE inhibitors were under patent and samples were available, the use of a month or 2 of samples to find the proper dose to control a particular patient's pressure was very helpful. In the current era, where the ACE inhibitors discussed here are inexpensive generics, that short-term advantage has faded. The advantage of a fixed-dose combination is that the patient only has to take 1 pill rather than 2. The disadvantage is that when 1 of the 2 agents needs to be titrated, a new combination preparation must be prescribed. If the patient requires a second titration, the process has to be repeated. Therefore, the most obvious use for fixed combinations like this is in a patient who has been well controlled on stable doses of both agents for some time.

While some practitioners may like to use this type of combination therapy as *initial* therapy in a particular patient who may need it (for instance, a patient whose blood pressure is > 20/10 mm Hg from the target), I recommend starting the ACE inhibitor and diuretic as separate preparations. The cost differential is negligible compared to the combination pill. The real advantage is that having the medications separate makes it much easier for you to titrate 1 of the agents, say the ACE inhibitor, by having the patient doubling up on the pills they already have without increasing the dose of the second agent simultaneously. Since we like to titrate the ACE inhibitor up to its maximum dose in complicated patients for protection against cardiovascular events (heart failure, coronary heart disease, adult-onset diabetes mellitus, etc), this approach allows us to maximize the ACE inhibitor protection while minimizing the side effects of the HCTZ, which are clearly dose dependent.

There are several fixed-dose combination products with an ACE inhibitor combined with a CCB. Tarka combines trandolapril with verapamil, Lexxel combines enalapril with felodopine, and Lotrel combines benazepril with amlodipine. These combinations have not been widely used, probably from the difficulty of titrating between the various combinations since all but Lexxel have multiple combinations available with different doses of each compound. There may be other ACE inhibitor combinations in the future, possibly combining an ACE inhibitor with an ARB or a different CCB.

Chapter 5
Calcium Channel Blockers

Calcium channel blockers, known as CCBs, have been widely used and very popular agents for blood pressure reduction. Their popularity with practitioners owes to their rapid and reliable reduction in blood pressure, their lack of potential for very serious side effects like angioedema, and their lack of negative metabolic effects like the electrolyte, glucose, or lipid effects seen with the thiazides. Recently, the most prominent of the dihydropyridines, amlodipine (Norvasc) and felodopine (Plendil) have become generic, making these agents much less expensive.

The CCBs, unlike other classes of antihypertensive agents, have 2 distinct subclasses of agents, with similar effectiveness but with significant differences between them. These molecular differences between the 2 subclasses lead to different mechanisms of action, along with different therapeutic uses and side effects. The non-dihydropyridines include diltiazem (Cardizem, Dilacor, and Tiazac) and verapamil (Calan, Covera, Isoptin, and Verelan). These agents differ chemically and in practice from the dihydropyridines, which include amlodipine (Norvasc), felodopine (Plendil), isradipine (Dynacirc), nicardipine (Cardene), and nifedipine GITS (Procardia XL and Adalat).

MECHANISM OF ACTION

Both subclasses of agents have a similar mechanism of action. They inhibit the intake of calcium ion influx into the vascular smooth muscle cell through the "slow channels" in the cell membrane. This lowers intracellular calcium ion concentration and dilates the smooth muscles. The difference between the classes comes from the specificity of the agents for smooth muscle sites affected. Diltiazem and verapamil are *nonspecific* in their actions. They therefore affect the central cardiac sites along with the peripheral vessel sites where the dihydropyridine CCBs have their effect. This cardiac effect for diltiazem and verapamil includes a negative ionotropic effect (reducing myocardial contractility), slowing heart rate (useful in tachycardia syndromes), and slowing conduction through the atrioventricular (AV) node (also useful in supraventricular tachycardia). These cardiac effects have therapeutic value, particularly in supraventricular tachycardia. However, they have negative potential, such as the induction of heart block at the AV node and worsening of reduced ejection fraction in patients with myocardial dysfunction. Therefore, before using these agents, prescribers should have a careful understanding of the patient's cardiac situation. They do remain, however, very useful in patients with atrial arrhythmias and hypertension.

The dihydropyridines do not have the potentially negative cardiac effects. Their only cardiac effect is to dilate the smooth muscles of the coronary arteries, making them very useful in the management of angina. They do *not* slow conduction through the AV node and they do *not* reduce myocardial contractility. Therefore, they can be used without concern in patients with myocardial dysfunction or AV node disease. This lack of serious side effects has propelled the dihydropyridines into a position of prominence in the management of hypertension.

Also, concern did emerge that the use of short-acting agents of this class may enhance myocardial problems, apparently from a rebound effect. Therefore, only the longer half-life agents, or the extended release products, should be used today. These longer half-life agents include the very popular amlodipine (Norvasc) and felodopine (Plendil).

The characteristics of the various agents are outlined in Table 5-1.

Table 5-1 Properties of the Calcium Channel Blockers

	Non-dihydropyridines	
Agents	**Daily Dose/Schedule**	**Cardiac Effects**
Diltiazem SR	120–360 mg/twice daily	↓BP, ↓SA node activity May ↓contractility
Diltiazem CD	120–360 mg/once daily	↓BP, ↓SA node activity May ↓contractility
Verapamil SR	120–360 mg/once daily	↓BP, ↓SA node activity May ↓contractility
	Dihydropyridines	
Amlodipine	2.5–10 mg daily	↓BP, ↓angina
Felodopine	2.5–10 mg daily	↓BP, ↓angina
Isradipine	2.5–10 mg twice daily	↓BP, ↓angina
Nicardipine	60–90 mg daily	↓BP, ↓angina
Nifedipine GITS	30–90 mg daily	↓BP, ↓angina

EVIDENCE OF EFFICACY

In contrast to the ACE inhibitors, which demonstrated efficacy at reducing cardiovascular events in a nearly complete variety of high-risk patients, the data for CCBs have not shown wide success in events reduction. These somewhat confusing and disappointing findings have led some to question where and when the CCBs should be used in the management of hypertension and cardiovascular disease.[74] I will attempt to summarize the trial data to make their usefulness clear.

In the most successful CCB trial to date, SYST-EUR, the dihydropyridine agent nitrendipine in doses of 10 to 40 mg/day was matched against placebo in elderly patients with isolated systolic hypertension.[15] Nitrendipine reduced stroke, major cardiovascular events, and cardiovascular mortality, with a trend for reduction in MI. These benefits were seen in patients treated only with nitrendipine and also in those treated with other agents added to the nitrendipine.[75] Nitrendipine showed trends toward a reduction in MI and the development of heart failure, but these did not reach statistical significance. These results were similar to those seen with thiazide diuretic use in the United States in the similar SHEP study.

Since CCBs were developed after many of the placebo-controlled trials had demonstrated that hypertension treatment was essential, further placebo-controlled studies are not available. There are, however, a series of trials and other analyses that have compared CCB therapy to other classes of agents.

Several trials have compared CCBs to traditional therapy with diuretics. Three compared dihydropyridine agents (felodopine or isradipine, nifedipine, and nicardipine), and 3 compared the non-dihydropyridine agents verapamil and diltiazem. The dihydropyridine trials showed equivalency with diuretics in preventing cardiovascular events, as did the non-dihydropyridine studies, which also had overall equivalency between the CCB and traditional treatments.[34,35,76] However, the verapamil and diltiazem studies had an interesting pattern, where the CCBs showed an increased potency for stroke reduction but a lessened potency for coronary heart disease reduction compared to the traditional treatments, while leading to an overall equivalency.[77]

A similar pattern was seen in several studies that utilized both ACE inhibitors and CCBs. In the STOP-2 trial, there were increased MIs but lower strokes in the CCB group.[78] Two other studies that compared verapamil versus a diuretic and/or atenolol failed to show any significant difference or pattern of difference.[79,80]

In studies looking at patients with cardiovascular on renal complications beyond hypertension, the differences with ACE inhibitors became more obvious. In 2 smaller studies with diabetic hypertensives, patients treated with ACE inhibitors had dramatically lower MI rates than patients treated with a dihydropyridine CCB.[67,81] In a final study comparing an ACE inhibitor to amlodipine in patients with hypertensive renal failure, the ACE inhibitor was superior to the dihydropyridine (amlodipine); it both slowed the renal deterioration and showed a trend for less MIs.[82] A similar pattern in comparison with ARBs was also seen. It could be argued that these other studies show the protective qualities of ACE inhibitors or ARBs and/or the lack of the protective qualities from the CCBs in complicated hypertensive patients, but these data do factor into consideration when deciding how and where to use CCB agents.

Further evidence indicates that the CCBs also do *not* have special efficacy in other cardiovascular complications frequently seen in hypertensive patients. In a study on the use of diltiazem after MI, diltiazem did not show overall positive benefit as a post-MI treatment.[83] A subsequent analysis showed that patients with systolic dysfunction (as ejection fraction of < 40%) fared *worse* on diltiazem.[84] This finding has led to recommendations that diltiazem (and possibly verapamil) not be used in patients with a decreased ejection fraction.[85] This concern spurred research into whether the dihydropyridine class also had this same effect. Several studies showed that the dihydropyridine class was *neutral* in heart failure patients, neither improving nor worsening their course.[86–88]

Finally, in patients with known atherosclerotic disease, amlodipine failed to slow the progression of atherosclerosis or to reduce clinical events, with the exception of angina or revascularization, over 36 months.[89]

Thus the scientific evidence on the potential for the CCBs is much more ambivalent than other classes, particularly the ACE inhibitors, ARBs, and beta-blockers. CCBs are very potent and easy-to-use antihypertensive agents. They can easily reduce elevated blood pressure and therefore reduce the cardiovascular complications of hypertension. However, they do not improve many of the complications of hypertension—MI, heart failure, or renal failure—once those problems have developed. Also, while they do not have the potential negative metabolic properties of the thiazides, they lack the MI protection of the ACE inhibitors seen in diabetic patients. Therefore, we need to consider all of these scientific facts as we identify the proper patient scenarios in which to use these potent and very popular agents.

AGENTS AND DOSAGE

In the non-dihydropyridine class of CCBs, diltiazem and verapamil are the agents available. Both agents have been available in generic formulation for many years, so they are both easily available and inexpensive. Also, both agents are now available in extended release preparations, which makes once-daily dosing much more acceptable for the patients. The dosage and agent information is summarized in Table 5-2.

For diltiazem, the traditional starting dose for hypertension is 120 mg once daily of the CD preparation, which is a once-daily preparation. Titration is done on a 7 to 14 day interval to allow for the appropriate blood pressure response. The traditional maximum dose for hypertension is 360 mg once daily. This is also the traditional maximum dose for angina management. Intravenous diltiazem is also used for the conversion of supraventricular tachyarrhythmias.

For verapamil, the extended release capsule, which is a once-daily preparation, has become the traditional preparation used in the management of hypertension. The traditional starting dose of the capsule is 240 mg once daily, with potential titration to 360 mg once daily after a week or more. The extended release tablet is a once- or twice-daily preparation, with initial doses of 180 to 240 mg administered once daily, and with increased doses of 180 to 240 mg administered twice daily (for total doses of 360–480 mg).

For the dihydropyridines, the doses are summarized in Table 5-2 also. All of the 5 preparations available in the United States are once-daily dosing, with the exception of isradipine, which is a twice daily.

SIDE EFFECTS

In general, the CCBs have a relatively low level of side effects, particularly the dihydropyridine group. For the dihydropyridine group, the side effects are mild and might be related to the smooth muscle relaxation, which is the mechanism for the lowering of blood pressure. The most common of these is pedal edema, which is relatively common but is *not* indicative of heart failure. Flushing, headache, and constipation are also seen. Again, these problems are mild and not indicative of systemic problems. They should not require alteration or cessation of therapy. The peripheral edema is dose related and is particularly noted at the maximal doses.

Gingival, or gum (periodontal), hyperplasia has been reported with all of the CCBs. The exact rate of occurrence is unclear because it was not assessed in the medical literature. A potential mechanism would be mediated through the smooth muscle relaxation seen with all of the agents. However, the exact relationship and rate of occurrence of this issue from the CCBs is unclear, but awareness of the potential for this issue is necessary.

With diltiazem and verapamil, there exists a potential for more serious side effects related to the suppression of conduction through the sinoatrial (SA) and atrioventricular (AV) nodes. This blockade of nodal activity can lead to minor findings like the development of first-degree AV block, but also to much more serious arrhythmia problems, especially if there is preexisting disease of the SA or particularly AV nodes. Caution is needed if verapamil is used in hypertrophic cardiomyopathy, where there are reports of second-degree or complete heart block, severe bradycardia, and even sudden death. Finally, both diltiazem and verapamil should be totally avoided in patients with heart failure or pulmonary congestion, particularly in the presence of active coronary artery disease because of the deleterious effect seen with diltiazem when it was studied in the patients in the post-MI study, especially in the patients with left ventricular dysfunction.

USE OF THE CCBs

With their excellent potency, low side effects, and ease of use, the dihydropyridine CCBs, most notably amlodipine, have been very widely used in all aspects of hypertension management. They are used as initial therapy or in conjunction with other agents. With their safety and tolerability, they are easy to use and well accepted by the patients.

However, they have not been able to match the ACE inhibitors, and even the ARBs, in offering specific protection against myocardial problems and the renal and cardiac protection seen with those agents in diabetes. Therefore, I would recommend that these agents should not be routine initial therapy in most hypertension patients. With the very high correlation between hypertension and metabolic syndrome and diabetes (most hypertensive patients are "pre-diabetic," if given enough time), I like to begin hypertension therapy with either an ACE inhibitor or an ARB—agents which have demonstrated protection for the hearts and kidneys of diabetic patients—as my traditional initial agents. This approach leads me to use dihydropyridine CCBs frequently but as a second or third agent on top of ACE inhibitor, ARB, or ACE/ARB therapy. The outstanding potency of the dihydropyridines make them very useful in controlling blood pressure in many patients, but the questions about their relative lack of cardiac protection, particularly in diabetics, positions them into secondary or tertiary use in many patients. There clearly is a group, namely elderly patients with predominantly systolic hypertension and no indication of metabolic syndrome (as shown in the SYST-EUR study), for whom the CCBs are excellent initial therapy, but other situations recommend other therapy initially.

Chapter 6

Angiotensin Receptor Blockers

The angiotensin receptor blockers, commonly called the ARBs, are one of the newer classes of antihypertensive agents. They were developed as antihypertensive agents, affecting the RAAS at a different location than the site of action of the ACE inhibitors. Since their introduction to the antihypertensive market, certain agents in the class have been shown to protect against diabetic renal disease, to treat heart failure, and to provide protection against recurrent cardiac problems in high-risk patients (like the benefit seen with ramipril, an ACE inhibitor, in the HOPE study).

They are, however, the only class of antihypertensive agents where well-conducted clinical trials have shown that there is a definable potency difference in lowering elevated blood pressure between the less potent original agents and the more potent newer agents. This is an important issue in practice because it means that data seen with one of the newer and very potent agents (like telmisartan in the recently completed ON-TARGET study) are not transferable to other agents in the class. Prescribers need to be aware of these potency differences and not assume, like we do with the ACE inhibitor class, that we can safely substitute one ARB for another. Therefore, we need to familiarize ourselves with the specific trials and use the agents based on the trials and the clinical result we expect to achieve.

MECHANISM OF ACTION

The ARBs work in the RAAS but in a different mechanism than do the ACE inhibitors. The ARBs block the binding of angiotensin II at the AT_1 receptors both directly at the vascular smooth muscle location and by blocking angiotensin II binding at the adrenal glands. The direct effect is that the blockade at the vascular smooth muscle at the periphery directly lowers the blood pressure, since angiotensin II is a potent vasoconstrictor agent. The inhibition of angiotensin II binding at the adrenal gland reduces the release of aldosterone, avoiding the retention of sodium and volume that is caused by aldosterone secretion, along with providing further lowering of the blood pressure systemically.

While the mechanisms for both the ARBs and the ACE inhibitors work in the renin angiotensin system, they work at different locations along the enzymatic pathway. These different sites of action do allow the 2 groups of agents, with caution (particularly toward the potential for potassium retention or deleterious renal effects) to be used together in the management of hypertension or heart failure. (See Figure 4-1.)

The exact mechanism of how the blockade of angiotensin II produces improvement in cardiovascular and renal problems is not exactly clear. The improvement in heart failure and recurrent cardiovascular events is most likely linked to reducing the vasoconstrictor effects of angiotensin II and the volume retention effects of excess aldosterone. The renal protective effects, like the benefits seen with the ACE inhibitors, are probably mediated through reducing increased pressure in the renal glomerulus by blocking the vasoconstrictor effects of angiotensin II.

The effectiveness in binding with the angiotensin II is the apparent explanation for the potency differences between the various agents in the ARB class. Comparator trials between various agents in the ARB class have been performed. They do show a clear difference in the potency of blood pressure lowering, with superior antihypertensive effects demonstrated with several of the newer ARBs when they were compared with the original ARBs, specifically losartan and valsartan. Direct comparison studies showed that irbesartan produced better blood pressure lowering than losartan, as monotherapy or when a diuretic was added.[90,91] Candesartan was also shown to have superior blood pressure lowering compared to losartan as monotherapy.[92] Telmisartan was shown to have increased blood pressure lowering compared to valsartan, either as monotherapy or when combined with diuretic.[93–95] Finally, olmesartan was shown to be more potent than losartan and valsartan, but not superior to irbesartan.[96]

This evidence sets up a very interesting situation. If we are only trying to control blood pressure, we can accommodate for these potency differences by monitoring the pressure and adjusting treatment. If a patient is on losartan or valsartan and is not well controlled, we could switch them to a more potent ARB, like telmisartan, candesartan, or irbesartan, rather than adding another additional agent. However, if we are also treating them for a complicating situation where a specific ARB has been proven to be effective, like candesartan in heart failure or telmisartan in high-risk coronary heart disease patients, then I think these particular situations mandate that we should use the agent and doses that were used in the specific studies.

EVIDENCE OF EFFICACY

As relative latecomers to the hypertension treatment spectrum, the ARBs have been comprehensively studied in a variety of cardiovascular and renal situations. I will present the pivotal studies categorized on the medical problem to be treated and attempt to explain how we should use the information to guide our practice.

Left Ventricular Hypertrophy

Hypertensive patients with left ventricular hypertrophy were evaluated in the LIFE study, which compared losartan-based treatment with atenolol-based treatment. Patients (9193 total) with hypertension and electrocardiogram (ECG) evidence of left ventricular hypertrophy were randomized to losartan or atenolol for 4 years. The degree of blood pressure control was equal between the 2 groups.[97] The composite endpoint of cardiovascular death, stroke, and MI was 13% lower in the losartan-based group, primarily due to lower cardiovascular mortality and a reduction in stroke in the losartan-treated group, while MI was not different. This is a difficult study to utilize now, since losartan has been shown to be one of the least potent of the ARBs at lowering blood pressure. Also, atenolol had not been shown to be cardioprotective in hypertension with left ventricular hypertrophy, so the positive effect of the losartan may be completely or partially due to the poor or nonexistent protection from atenolol.

Recent Myocardial Infarction

In patients with recent MI, several studies were undertaken to see if ARBs had the same protective properties as had been shown with ACE inhibitors. In OPTIMAAL, losartan was compared to captopril in 5477 patients with recent acute MI and evidence of left ventricular dysfunction who were randomized to captopril or losartan and followed for nearly 3 years.[98] The endpoint of total mortality showed a non-significant trend in favor of captopril, leading the authors to conclude that ACE inhibitor treatment should remain the initial choice in this situation. A similar study was VALIANT, which compared valsartan, captopril, or a combination of both in patients with recent MI and left ventricular dysfunction.[99] This study enrolled over 12,000 patients and ran for 2 years. It showed *equivalency* between valsartan monotherapy, captopril monotherapy, and combined valsartan/captopril therapy in all of the endpoints of mortality and cardiovascular events. Therefore, valsartan was equal to captopril in patients with recent MI and left ventricular dysfunction, but adding the 2 together did not increase the benefit.

Chronic Heart Failure

In patients with chronic heart failure, there has been extensive research on several ARBs. The earliest work was on losartan, where a preliminary study, ELITE I, suggested that losartan had a trend toward lower mortality in patients with stable heart failure compared with captopril.[100] When this study was repeated in ELITE II, different results were seen. ELITE II randomized 3152 patients with stable heart failure to losartan (50 mg daily) or to captopril (50 mg, 3 times a day) for nearly 2 years. Total mortality and sudden death both showed a non-significant trend favoring captopril, reinforcing the value of ACE inhibitors in heart failure.[101]

The Val-HeFT study compared valsartan (160 mg twice daily) with placebo in patients with chronic heart failure. Val-HeFT is a complicated and difficult study to evaluate. Most, but not all, patients were already on ACE inhibitor therapy, but only 35% were on beta-blockers. There was no difference in mortality between the valsartan and placebo groups. There was an improvement in the combined endpoint of mortality and morbidity, primarily driven by a reduction in hospital admissions for heart failure.[102] The most difficult data were based on the other heart failure therapy that the patients were taking. Most of the benefit was in the subset of patients who were not on either an ACE inhibitor or beta-blocker. Indeed, in the group on *both* ACE inhibitor and beta-blocker, valsartan had an *adverse* effect on mortality. Therefore, it is difficult to define how, if at all, valsartan should be used in the heart failure population.

The CHARM study, in contrast, offers a much clearer picture of how to use an ARB in heart failure. CHARM was a combination of 3 efforts in patients with heart failure, (1) using candesartan *added* to patients on ACE inhibitor therapy (CHARM added), (2) using candesartan in patients *intolerant* of ACE inhibitor therapy (CHARM alternative), and (3) using candesartan in patients with heart failure and an ejection fraction of > 40% (CHARM preserved).[103] In CHARM added, the addition of candesartan to patients with heart failure already on ACE inhibitor therapy reduced cardiovascular death and hospital admissions when compared to placebo in heart failure patients already on ACE inhibitor therapy.[104] CHARM alternative showed that ACE inhibitor-intolerant patients with heart failure placed on candesartan had reduced cardiovascular death or hospitalizations versus those on placebo.[105] CHARM preserved, with heart failure patients with an ejection fraction of > 40%, had no effect on mortality but showed a reduction in hospitalizations for heart failure in patients on candesartan when compared to patients on placebo.[106] Taken in whole, these studies showed that candesartan improved functioning and events in heart failure patients, the clearest evidence for any of the ARBs in this most serious condition. This type of treatment needs to be administered cautiously, with an initial dose of 4 mg daily and with gradual titration every 2 weeks toward the 32 mg target dose. Careful monitoring of blood pressure and serum potassium and renal function are also necessary, but the evidence is promising.

High-Risk Patients

The use of an ARB in high-risk patients was studied in the ON-TARGET study. ON-TARGET studied 23,000 patients with previous vascular disease (MI, CVA, and PVD) or with diabetes with end organ damage. They were randomized to telmisartan 80 mg/day, ramipril 10 mg/day, or both, and they were followed for nearly 5 years. There was no difference in the primary endpoint between the 3 groups. A particularly important finding was that the patients on telmisartan had the same level of cardiac events as those on ramipril, showing that telmisartan was equivalent to ramipril in protecting against subsequent cardiovascular events in these high-risk patients. However, the combination therapy group, randomized to *both* telmisartan and ramipril together, did not have any enhanced protection from cardiac events compared to the patients on telmisartan or ramipril alone. These patients on a combination of both telmisartan and ramipril together *did* have an increased amount of hypotension, syncope, and renal dysfunction, so caution and careful monitoring is important when an ACE inhibitor and ARB are used together.[107]

This study is extremely important, since it shows that telmisartan 80 mg offers the same degree of cardiovascular protection that ramipril 10 mg offered in the pivotal HOPE study.

Table 6-1 Special Indications for ARB therapy

Indication	ARB	Doses	Effects	Caution
HBP with LVH	Losartan	50–100 mg	↓death, ↓CVA	
Heart Failure w/o ACE-I Therapy	Candesartan Valsartan	4–32 mg 40–160 mg twice daily	↓CV death, ↓MI, ↓HF ↓HF	↓BP, ↑K+, ↑creat. ↓BP, ↑K+, ↑creat.
Heart Failure with ACE Therapy	Candesartan	4–32 mg	↓CV death, ↓MI, ↓HF	↓BP, ↑K+, ↑creat.
High Risk for CVD w/o ACE	Telmisartan	40–80 mg	↓All CVD events	↓BP, ↑creat.
AODM with Renal Disease	Losartan Irbesartan	50–100 mg 150–300 mg	↓renal decline, ↓proteinuria	↑K+.

Therefore, if high-risk patients are unable to tolerate an ACE inhibitor because of cough or angioedema, telmisartan will confer the same degree of long-term protection. The fact that combination therapy offered increased side effects without extra benefit is also very important. This study was followed by the TRANSCEND study, which used telmisartan versus placebo in high-risk patients like those in the HOPE study but who were intolerant of ACE inhibitor therapy. The results were not as conclusive, with a non-significant trend of reduced events in the telmisartan group, which was due to the addition of an "admission for heart failure" to the composite primary endpoint.[108] When they looked at only the endpoints used in the HOPE study, the results were significantly improved.

Finally, several of the ARBs have been shown to protect kidney function, in both diabetic renal disease and non-diabetic renal disease.[109–111] These studies show that use of ARBs slows or reduces renal decline across the spectrum of causes of renal problems, not just in the diabetic renal disease where the benefit was first documented.[112,113] Therefore, therapy with either an ACE inhibitor or an ARB is standard care in diabetic and non-diabetic renal disease.

A summary of the agents and the indication for ARBs in special patient situations is provided in Table 6-1.

AGENTS AND DOSAGE

There are currently 7 ARBs on the market, with other agents in development. The 7 agents and their traditional hypertension doses are listed in Table 6-2.

Similarly to the ACE inhibitors, the action of the ARBs through the renin-angiotensin system means that their effectiveness in lowering blood pressure is enhanced by combining them with a thiazide diuretic. Therefore, 6 of the 7 marketed ARBs have preparations combined with HCTZ available in combination form. Only eprosartan (Teveten) does not have a combination

Table 6-2 Angiotensin Receptor Blockers (ARBs)

Agent	Doses	Dosing Schedule
Candesartan (*Atacand*)	16–32 mg	Once daily
Eprosartan (*Teveten*)	400–600 mg	Once or twice daily (400 mg twice daily maximum)
Irbesartan (*Avapro*)	150–300 mg	Once daily
Losartan (*Cozaar*)	50–100 mg	Once or twice daily (maximum 50 mg twice daily)
Olmesartan (*Benicar*)	40–80 mg	Once daily
Telmisartan (*Micardis*)	40–80 mg	Once daily
Valsartan (*Diovan*)	80, 160, or 320 mg	Once daily

Table 6-3 ARB and HCTZ Combination Products

Agent Combinations	Doses Available
Candesartan/HCTZ (*Atacand HCT*)	16/12.5 mg, 32/12.5 mg
Irbesartan/HCTZ (*Avalide*)	150/12.5 mg, 300/12.5 mg, 300/25 mg
Losartan/HCTZ (*Hyzaar*)	50/12.5 mg, 100/12.5 mg, 100/25 mg
Olmesartan/HCTZ (*Benicar HCT*)	20/12.5 mg, 40/12.5 mg, 40/25 mg
Telmisartan/HCTZ (*Micardis HCT*)	40/12.5 mg, 80/12.5 mg, 80/25 mg
Valsartan/HCTZ (*Diovan HCT*)	80/12.5 mg, 160/12.5 mg, 160/25 mg, 320/12.5 mg, 320/25 mg

product. The various combination products are listed in Table 6-3. These products are used *only* in hypertension, and they are all dosed once daily.

As you can see in Table 6-3, the dosing spectrum for these agents in hypertension is quite simple, with most agents only having 1 initial dose and a maximum dose for 1 titration step. Traditional therapy is to start at the traditional starting dose and then to titrate, if necessary, to the maximum dose. It is very common to use diuretic combination therapy with the ARBs. An ARB/HCTZ combination can be used as initial therapy in a person whose blood pressure elevation requires 2-drug therapy as initial therapy, with a blood pressure > 20/10 above target levels. The ARB/HCTZ combinations are particularly useful in African American patients, who are often very responsive to diuretic therapy, and in elderly patients, who often require diuretic therapy due to resistant systolic pressures. In general, to reduce the diuretic side effects, I try to use the lowest diuretic dose available, recognizing that in some patients we will have to go to the maximum dose.

SIDE EFFECTS

In general, the great attractiveness of the ARB class of agents is its extremely low rate of side effects. In uncomplicated hypertension, their level of side effects is usually comparable to, or lower than, the placebo patients in the clinical trials. They do not cause any of the traditional antihypertensive side effects like fatigue, malaise, sexual dysfunction, or electrolyte problems. They reduce the rate of development of diabetes in many studies and protect against diabetic renal disease. They require minimal monitoring, particularly when used in monotherapy (periodic evaluation of renal function is warranted).

Because of their low level of side effects, many practitioners use an ARB in combination with an ACE inhibitor for management of hypertension *not yet complicated* by heart failure, cardiovascular disease, or renal disease. This combination is very well tolerated and generally quite safe, but it does require more careful monitoring of serum potassium and creatinine.

Because their effectiveness is moderated through the RAAS, ARBs (like ACE inhibitors) should not be used in pregnant females due to fetal injury potential. Therefore, I would avoid, if at all possible, using an ARB (or an ACE inhibitor) in a fertile female.

USE OF THE ARBs

The ARBs are becoming premier agents, like the ACE inhibitors, in the management of hypertension and cardiovascular disease. Because of their nearly complete absence of side effects, they are excellent initial or supplemental agents for the management of the uncomplicated hypertensive patient.

What is exciting, but requires careful attention to the research details, is the emerging data in *complicated* cardiovascular disease. Some of the ARBs have proven success in the management of cardiovascular disease, and they should be used appropriately—telmisartan in ACE inhibitor-intolerant high-risk cardiovascular disease patients, candesartan in heart failure patients with or without ACE inhibitor therapy (also valsartan in such patients), and irbesartan or losartan in diabetic renal disease patients. We should feel comfortable going to these agents early in the development of hypertension, with the hope that aggressive management with these agents could avoid these issues in the future.

Chapter 7
Beta-Blockers

Beta-blockers have been one of the mainstays of the management of hypertension and other forms of cardiovascular disease for several decades. Beta-blockers were identified as "preferential" initial therapy in the JNC-IV report quite some time ago. However, in a careful examination of the data, many have begun to challenge that recommendation for using beta-blockers as initial therapy.

Beta-blockers work by inhibiting the beta-adrenergic or catecholamine (sympathetic) system. The catecholamine system is widespread throughout the body and is influenced both by the systemic release of epinephrine and norepinephrine, along with an extensive intracellular beta-adrenergic system. Because of the extensive nature of this system, the physiologic effects of the stimulation of this system are widespread, affecting the cardiac system (increased vascular contractility, increased heart rate and contractility, and, therefore, increased myocardial oxygen demand), the pulmonary system (increased bronchodilation), the metabolic system (increased insulin secretion, increased gluconeogenesis, and increased glycogenolysis), and activation of the RAAS through renin release.

MECHANISMS OF ACTION

The beta-adrenergic system is located in a wide variety of tissues throughout the body; thus the beta-blockers have diffuse effects in many systems other than the cardiac system.

The beta-blockers exert their effect by binding at the beta-adrenergic binding sites and inhibiting the simulative properties of the catecholamine hormones. These beta receptors are in 2 subtypes, the beta-1 receptors, which are located in the cardiac tissues, and the beta-2 receptors, which are located in the pulmonary and other non-cardiac tissues. There are several classes of beta-blockers, with many of them having a preference for *all* of the beta-1 and beta-2 receptors ("non-selective") and others having a preference for the cardiac beta-1 receptors ("cardiac-selective"). The cardiac selectivity is a "relative" selectivity that appears to diminish or disappear at higher doses, casting doubts that cardiac selectivity is of a real and clinically important significance. The assumption that the cardiac-selective beta-blockers would have less pulmonary and other side effects has never been substantiated scientifically.

Secondly, there are agents, pindolol and acebutolol, that have an additional property of mild agonist properties at the beta-2 receptors. The theory behind these agents is that they can lower blood pressure with less reduction of cardiac output and less bradycardia. Whether these theoretical properties have clinical significance is unproven, and these agents have *not* been shown to reduce cardiac events like the traditional agents. Finally, 2 of the beta-blockers, labetolol (Normodyne, Trandate) and carvedilol (Coreg), have some inhibition of the peripheral alpha-adrenergic system in addition to their beta-blockade. It is also unclear whether this modest secondary effect has significant additional benefit.

EVIDENCE OF EFFICACY

Despite how long the beta-blockers have been recommended for and utilized in the treatment of hypertension, we do not have the clear proof of efficacy in reducing cardiovascular events in the treatment of uncomplicated hypertension that we see with diuretics. Beta-blockers were actually used as secondary therapy, added on to thiazide therapy as pressures necessitated, in the early pivotal trials. These trials included the HAPPHY, MAPHY, and MRC elderly trials.[54,114,115] However, in the MRC elderly study, atenolol did not reduce events compared to placebo, while diuretic-based treatment did reduce events.[54] Several more recent studies have raised similar questions. In the previously mentioned LIFE study, patients with left ventricular hypertrophy and hypertension had better events reduction on losartan, an ARB, than on the beta-blocker atenolol.[97] Similarly, in the ASCOT-BPLA trial, patients on an atenolol/diuretic-based treatment had more cardiovascular events than patients on a CCB/ACE inhibitor regimen.[40]

Several comprehensive reviews have also challenged the routine use of beta-blocker as initial therapy in hypertension. A review by Messerli and colleagues in 1998 evaluated the beta-blocker trials and stated that, in contrast to diuretics, beta-blockers had *not* been proven to reduce cardiovascular events in hypertension treatment and should no longer be recommended as first-line therapy.[116] A second review found that, while beta-blockers reduced stroke in hypertension patients, they did not reduce death or MI. This analysis also noted an increased potential to develop new onset diabetes in hypertensive patients assigned to beta-blockers.[117]

While there are reasonable questions about the efficacy of beta-blockers as initial therapy in *uncomplicated* hypertension, there is overwhelming evidence for their power in preventing recurrent cardiac events and mortality in patients with MI or heart failure.

Beginning in 1981, beta-blockade after MI showed a dramatic reduction in death and recurrent MI in initial studies with timolol and the following year with propranolol.[118,119] Follow-up studies showed that this protection was seen with many of the beta-blocker preparations. A number of agents have been shown to reduce the number and severity of supraventricular and ventricular arrhythmias. Beta-blockers have been shown to reduce angina symptoms and also to be therapeutic in the management of hypertrophic cardiomyopathy. Finally, 2 preparations available in the United States have been shown to reduce cardiac events and mortality in heart failure patients. Extended release metoprolol (Toprol XL, 100–200 mg) and carvedilol (Coreg, 25 mg twice daily) appear to be equally efficacious in this most serious disorder.[43,44] Interestingly, a different beta-blocker, bucindolol, did not prove efficacious in heart failure.[46] This finding leads to the recommendation that we should use the beta-blockers and the doses used in the studies to treat this most serious and frequently fatal condition. This recommendation was underscored by the COMET trial, which compared proven heart failure doses of carvedilol against smaller doses of immediate release metoprolol twice daily.[43] The superiority of carvedilol in this study emphasizes that we should use only the studied doses of extended release metoprolol (100–200 mg/day) or carvedilol (12.5 or 25 mg twice daily).

In addition, beta-blockers have been studied and found to be very useful in problems outside of the cardiovascular system. These conditions include prophylaxis for migraine and other vascular headaches, for essential tremor, for the management of endocrine disorders including thyrotoxicosis and pheochromocytoma, and for mitral valve prolapse syndrome and the anxiety symptoms that are part of the syndrome.

AGENTS AND DOSAGE

Currently, there are 16 systemic beta-blockers on the US market. Most of these have been on the market for many years and are now low-cost generics. Recently, a new beta-blocker, nebivolol (Bystolic), has come onto the US market. The agents and their traditional doses are listed in Table 7-1. Fifteen of these agents, excluding only sotalol (Betapace), are approved and were originally marketed for the treatment of hypertension. Sotalol has been developed and utilized as an antiarrhythmic agent, even though it does have antihypertensive and antianginal properties. Carvedilol (Coreg) is a beta-blocker that also has alpha-blockade properties. It is utilized primarily as treatment for heart failure, even though it is effective in hypertension and in post-MI patients.

Table 7-1 Beta-Blockers

Agent	Doses	Dosing Schedule	Indications
Acebutolol	200–400 mg 300–400 mg	Twice daily Twice daily	Hypertension, arrhythmia
Atenolol	50–200 mg	Once daily	HBP, angina, post-MI
Betaxolol	10–20 mg	Once daily	Hypertension
Bisoprolol	5–10 mg	Once daily	Hypertension
Carteolol	2.5–10 mg	Once daily	Hypertension
Carvedilol (Coreg)	3.125 titrated up to 25 mg	Twice daily	Heart failure, HBP, post-MI
[a]Labetalol	100–400 mg	Twice daily	Hypertension
Metoprolol	50–200 mg	Twice daily	Hypertension, angina, post-MI
Metoprolol extended release	50–400 mg	Once daily	HBP, angina, post-MI, heart failure
Nadolol	40–320 mg	Once daily	Hypertension, angina
Nebivolol (Bystolic)	5–40 mg	Once daily	Hypertension
Oxprenolol	20–80 mg	Three times/day	Hypertension
Penbutolol	20 mg	Once daily	Hypertension
Pindolol	5–30 mg	Twice daily	Hypertension
[b]Propranolol	40–120 mg	Twice daily	Hypertension, angina, post-MI
Extended release propranolol	80–640 mg	Once daily	Hypertension, angina, post-MI
Sotalol	80–160 mg	Twice daily	Arrhythmia
Timolol	10–20 mg	Twice daily	HBP, post-MI

[a]Intravenous dose available.
[b]Intravenous and oral solution available.

There are currently 6 beta-blocker/thiazide combination preparations on the US market. These products are for use in treating hypertension. The combination products and their doses are listed in Table 7-2.

Table 7-2 Beta-Blocker/Diuretic Combinations

Agents	Combination Doses
Atenolol/chlorthalidone	50/25 mg, 100/25 mg
Bisoprolol/HCTZ	2.5/6.25 mg, 5/6.25 mg, 10/6.25 mg
Metoprolol/HCTZ	50/25 mg, 100/25 mg
Nadolol/bendroflumethiazide	40/5 mg, 80/5 mg
Propranolol-LA/HCTZ	40/25 mg, 80/25 mg
Timolol/HCTZ	10/25 mg

SIDE EFFECTS

The amount and severity of side effects seen with beta-blockers remain the major restriction on their use. The side effects include both symptomatic problems like fatigue and sexual dysfunction, along with metabolic effects.

Common Side Effects

The more common side effects are systemic and appear to be principally mediated through the central nervous system (CNS). These symptoms include dizziness/lightheadedness, fatigue, mental depression, bizarre dreams, and sexual dysfunction. While some of these symptoms, particularly fatigue, could be mediated through decreased cardiac output from bradycardia and decreased cardiac ionotropic effects, the symptoms are probably mediated through the central nervous system instead. Since these side effects increase with higher doses and may be more prominent with agents with a higher lipid solubility (which would lead to higher penetration of the CNS), these effects are predominantly mediated centrally. These side effects can be difficult in a patient requiring a beta-blocker, such as a patient with heart failure or coronary artery disease. However, we can make product selections to help reduce this complication. I avoid propranolol because its high lipid solubility appears to make these symptoms more prominent. Also, by using the extended release metoprolol, which produces a lower but more consistent serum level, I can usually achieve the therapeutic dose of at least 100 mg/day in most patients without significant CNS side effects.

Cardiac Side Effects

Beta-blockers can produce specific cardiac side effects, including bradycardia and increased AV heart block, so caution should be maintained when patients have these preexisting problems. The bradycardia and decreased cardiac output can worsen peripheral circulation symptoms, particularly in patients with Raynaud's phenomenon or peripheral artery disease. A beta-blocker with ISA (intrinsic sympathomimetic activity), including acebutolol, penbutolol, pindolol, or labetolol, may produce less bradycardia or reduced cardiac output, though this is not proven.

Pulmonary Side Effects

Bronchospasm, particularly in asthmatic patients with classical reactive airway disease, may be initiated or exacerbated by beta-blockers. Therefore, beta-blockers should be avoided in patients with asthma, particularly in asthmatic patients with significant reactive airway disease. It is much less clear in chronic obstructive pulmonary disease (COPD) patients, many of whom have only a very limited amount of reactive airway disease. Patients with COPD frequently also have coronary artery disease, heart failure, or both—conditions where the use of beta-blockers can be very beneficial. In general, asthma is a contraindication to beta-blocker therapy. Emphysema, or COPD, is a condition that requires caution when using beta-blockers, and there are patients in whom it might be advisable to obtain pulmonary function tests to determine if they have enough reactive airway disease that would discourage you from cautiously using beta-blockers.

Metabolic Side Effects

Metabolic abnormalities are common with beta-blockers. In general, the beta-blockers have modest negative effects on serum lipid levels, increasing total cholesterol, low-density lipoprotein cholesterol, and triglycerides, in addition to lowering high-density lipoprotein cholesterol.[120] These changes are diminished or absent with the beta-blockers with ISA. The clinical significance of these changes in the current era, where highly potent statin therapy can easily alter lipid values, is probably quite limited. There has long been concern about whether beta-blocker therapy might reduce the hypoglycemic response of catecholamine release, including tremor, tachycardia, and sweating. Therefore, beta-blockers need to be used cautiously in insulin-dependent diabetic patients. Since many diabetic patients have coronary artery disease and heart failure, careful use and gentle titration of beta-blockers often may be necessary in these patients.

USE OF THE BETA-BLOCKERS

Use of beta-blockers in hypertension has evolved over the decades. With the introduction of highly potent agents with very good side effect profiles, like the ACE inhibitors, ARBs, and CCBs, routine beta-blocker use as initial therapy for hypertension has declined. Given the questions about the efficacy of beta-blocker therapy previously discussed, it is time that beta-blockers become secondary, rather than primary agents in hypertension. By secondary, I mean they should be reserved as additional agents in patients who are already on several blood pressure lowering agents without achieving complete control. Also, there are several *critical conditions*, like heart failure and coronary artery disease, where their use is mandatory (unless clearly contraindicated). Since there are millions of patients with heart failure and/or coronary artery disease that need beta-blockers, they will remain commonly used agents, even as their early use in uncomplicated hypertension declines.

Chapter 8
Alpha-1 Blockers

The alpha-1 blockers are agents that lower blood pressure by reducing smooth muscle tone at the periphery. They have not enjoyed particular success, and they are rarely employed any more as initial therapy agents as monotherapy for hypertension. They have modest blood pressure lowering effects and a significant side effect profile, a combination that has limited their usage in the broad hypertension market.

Interestingly, after they had gone to market as antihypertensive agents, it was discovered that the smooth muscle relaxation properties produced by blocking the alpha-1 receptor also had a therapeutic benefit in men with symptoms of benign prostatic hyperplasia (BPH). How much of the current alpha-1 blocker use is for hypertension alone, how much is for symptomatic BPH, and how much is for both problems in male patients is impossible to determine. However, the potential for benefit for both problems with 1 inexpensive medication is an important characteristic to remember.

MECHANISM OF ACTION

The alpha-1 blockers work at the periphery. Their mechanism is mediated through the postsynaptic receptor of the sympathetic nervous system. In this system, the sympathetic nervous system stimulates vasoconstriction through the smooth muscles responsible for the tone around the vascular system. The sympathetic nervous system mediates this vascular tone by releasing norepinephrine from the presynaptic junction. This norepinephrine migrates to the postsynaptic junction and binds on the alpha-1 receptors, increasing the smooth muscle contraction. The alpha-1 blockers bind competitively at the alpha-1 binding sites on the postsynaptic junction. This blocks access to the binding sites for the norepinephrine and relaxes the muscle tone around the vessels, thereby lowering vascular tone and blood pressure.

This effect is also responsible for the reduction of BPH symptoms with alpha-1 blockers. In fact, the symptoms of BPH are not caused by the size of the prostate, but by the smooth muscle tone in the lower bladder, prostatic urethra, and urethra. The alpha-1 blockers reduce this enhanced smooth muscle tone by the mechanism described previously. This reduction in smooth muscle tone gives significant and rapid relief in BPH symptoms. The reduction in tone can reduce BPH symptoms within a week of reaching the therapeutic dose of alpha-1 blocker.

This mechanism is also responsible for one of the most visible side effects of alpha-1 blockers, peripheral or pedal edema.

EVIDENCE OF EFFICACY

Unlike the agents in the previous chapters, the alpha-1 blockers do not have a pattern of solid scientific evidence of reducing cardiovascular events in hypertension patients. This absence of data, along with their side effect profile, has relegated the alpha-1 blockers to a very limited role in hypertension treatment and in the hypertension guidelines.

The only clear events trial was a comparison against chlorthalidone in the difficult-to-evaluate ALLHAT trial. In ALLHAT, hypertensive patients were assigned to treatment with 1 of 4 treatment arms: chlorthalidone (diuretic), doxazosin (alpha-1 blocker), amlodipine (CCB), or lisinopril (ACE inhibitor). The doxazosin arm was stopped early for safety reasons. The primary endpoint of the trial, fatal or nonfatal MI, was not different between chlorthalidone and doxazosin.[121] However, the doxazosin arm had a higher rate of secondary endpoints, particularly driven by a much higher rate of heart failure, but also for angina and stroke. It is difficult to interpret these findings since heart failure was diagnosed clinically and could have been overdiagnosed from pedal edema seen as a doxazosin side effect. Also, the doxazosin group had slightly higher systolic blood pressure, which could have accounted for the increased stroke results.

This study resulted in many guidelines (and practitioners) dropping alpha-1 blockers from the list of recommended (or used) first-line agents.[30] I agree with that recommendation and practice, but I do think alpha-1 blockers have a role in third-line therapy in difficult-to-control patients and for those male patients with difficult-to-control blood pressure and symptoms of BPH. A further sub-analysis of the ASCOT-BPLA hypertension study did use doxazosin as third-line therapy in the step titration of the trial.[122] That study found that doxazosin was an effective third-step agent in the trial. It produced reasonable reduction in both systolic and diastolic pressure (−11.7/6.9 mm Hg), it did not have excess heart failure or other cardiac events, and it had a favorable effect on lipid parameters.

A series of trials evaluating both terazosin and doxazosin has been conducted in men with symptomatic BPH. These trials have enrolled men with elevated blood pressure and with normal (or controlled) blood pressure. Both terazosin and doxazosin reduced BPH symptoms by more than 50%.[123,124] These studies also gave very clear and important evidence about the blood pressure effect when alpha-1 blockers are used to treat symptomatic BPH. In men who had elevated blood pressure at the entry into the trials, there was a significant reduction in blood pressure.

Table 8-1 Alpha-1 Blockers

Agent	Initial Dose	Schedule	Titration Steps (if necessary)
Doxazosin	1 mg (one week)	Daily (bedtime)	2 mg for 1 week 4 mg 1–2 weeks 8 mg 1–2 weeks 16 mg
Terazosin	1 mg (2–3 days)	Daily (bedtime)	2 mg for 1–2 weeks 5 mg for 1–2 weeks 10 mg

However, if the entry blood pressure was either normal or was controlled by medication, the blood pressure reduction from terazosin or doxazosin was small and clinically insignificant. Therefore, these agents are useful for treating symptomatic BPH regardless of the blood pressure.

AGENTS AND DOSAGE

Three alpha-1 blockers are currently available in the United States. They are listed with their dose ranges in Table 8-1. Even though prazosin is still available, its short half-life and 3 times a day dosing means there is no reason to use it at this time. Both doxazosin and terazosin have longer half-lives that allow for once-daily dosing.

Because of the tendency of these agents to cause dizziness and lightheadedness, I recommend administering them at bedtime as a once-daily dose of doxazosin or terazosin. These agents have the potential to cause a "first dose orthostatic hypotension" syndrome, so they need to be started at the sub-therapeutic 1 mg dose of either doxazosin or terazosin. They should then be titrated gradually, usually about every 1 to 2 weeks, up through the therapeutic doses until reaching the desired control or the maximum dose (10 mg of terazosin or 16 mg of doxazosin). Very importantly, if the patient stops the agent or misses even a single dose, the titration must be begun again at the 1 mg dose. Restarting or initiating therapy above the 1 mg dose can lead to significant chest pain and other symptoms.

SIDE EFFECTS

The side effect profiles of the alpha-1 blockers are noticeable and do restrict their use. The risk of postural or orthostatic hypotension, even with syncope, is an uncommon but possible side effect. In our large population-based BPH study, orthostatic dizziness was seen in 2% and postural hypotension in 1% of patients.[124] It is most risky in older men getting out of bed at night or in the morning, but it can happen at any time.

Other side effects are more common but are difficult to define, including dizziness, fatigue, somnolence, pedal edema, and palpitations. The rates of these symptoms are not clearly defined, but symptoms are reported in about 10% to 15% of patients in studies.[124] Rates in practice may be different. My own experience when using these agents in men with BPH taking a bedtime dose is that they rarely report symptoms. However, proper attention to caution about and inquiry for symptoms is important.

USE OF THE ALPHA-1 BLOCKERS

The alpha-1 blockers have a limited, but important place in the management of hypertension. As outlined, they are not appropriate initial or even second-step agents. They do have a place, albeit somewhat limited, as additive agents onto several other agents, in very difficult-to-control hypertension patients. They do require a well organized and compliant patient to avoid missed doses and the need to reinstitute titration from the starting dose.

Their truly beneficial function is in a male, with or without hypertension, with symptomatic BPH. Both doxazosin and terazosin are effective and well tolerated in this common and uncomfortable condition.

Chapter 9

Renin Inhibitors

Recently we have seen a new class of agent introduced for the management of hypertension, a renin inhibitor. Aliskiren (Tekturna) directly inhibits renin, resulting in a decrease of plasma renin activity. This decrease in plasma renin activity inhibits the conversion of angiotensinogen to angiotensin I, which subsequently reduces the formation of angiotensin II, which is a potent vasoconstrictor. Lowering angiotensin II production reduces blood pressure. (See Figure 4-1.) Aliskiren reduces plasma renin activity by about 50% to 80%.[125] It is unknown if there are other mechanisms affecting blood pressure that are involved with aliskiren therapy.

EVIDENCE OF EFFICACY

Because of its newness on the market, aliskiren has not been studied in any trial, either for hypertension or other cardiovascular disorders, to see if it will reduce cardiovascular events like the ACE inhibitors, diuretics, and other classes. Aliskiren has been studied as monotherapy in uncomplicated hypertension patients, with reductions of both systolic and diastolic pressures comparable to other classes of agents. Aliskiren has been studied in combination with HCTZ with blood pressure reductions similar to other HCTZ combination therapies. It has also been studied in combination the ARB valsartan (Diovan), with blood pressure reductions comparable to what has been seen with other ARB combinations. Aliskiren has not been studied in combination with ACE inhibitors or CCBs.

AGENTS AND DOSAGE

Aliskiren is currently the only renin inhibitor on the market. It is marketed in 2 doses, 150 mg and 300 mg, each to be given once daily.

SIDE EFFECTS

The side effect pattern for aliskiren is reasonable and modest. Like all agents that affect the RAAS, it should not be used in pregnancy, or even in fertile females. There have been rare reports of angioedema, as seen with the ACE inhibitors.

Aliskiren has not been studied in patients with impaired renal function, so caution should be used if considering aliskiren in this population. Hyperkalemia was rare in aliskiren monotherapy (< 1%), but higher rates should be expected in combination with an ACE inhibitor in a diabetic population. Therefore, routine monitoring of electrolytes is in order.[125]

Other less severe side effects appear to be mild and self-limited, like gastrointestinal distress, diarrhea, and a slight increase in cough.

USE OF THE RENIN INHIBITOR

Aliskiren appears to be a reasonable antihypertensive agent, with reasonable efficacy and safety. Without any long-term events reduction data, it is difficult to define a clear patient situation where it will be particularly useful, either in combination with or instead of the other very well defined antihypertensive agents.

Chapter 10

Aldosterone Receptor Blockers

Another relatively new product is eplerenone (Inspra), an aldosterone receptor blocker.

MECHANISM OF ACTION

Eplerenone binds to the mineralocorticoid receptor site where aldosterone binds. Thus, eplerenone inhibits the effect of aldosterone by blocking its binding site. The consequent reductions in aldosterone's vasoconstrictor effect and in its sodium and water retention effect result in lowered blood pressure. (See Figure 4-1.)

EVIDENCE OF EFFICACY

Eplerenone has been studied in a very extensive trial in patients with heart failure in the post-MI situation. In that study, called EPHESUS, eplerenone was studied versus placebo in post-MI patients with heart failure or left ventricular dysfunction, with patients receiving optimal medical therapy, including ACE inhibitors, ARBs, diuretics, and beta-blockers. Patients receiving eplerenone had a significant reduction in total mortality, driven primarily by a reduction in cardiac mortality, and with a reduction in hospitalizations for cardiovascular causes.[126]

In hypertension, however, eplerenone was studied as monotherapy and in combinations with other agents. The systolic and diastolic reductions were comparable with the reductions seen with other therapies. They do not report specific combination trials with particular products, but they do report that the blood pressure reductions seen with the combinations are those that would be expected.

AGENTS AND DOSAGE

For hypertension, eplerenone is begun at 50 mg once daily, with a possible dose titration to 50 mg twice daily after 2 to 4 weeks. For heart failure, the initial dose is 25 mg once daily, with a titration to 50 mg once daily within 4 weeks. Heart failure is *not* treated at a dose greater than 50 mg *once daily*. Patients with a serum creatinine > 2.0 mg/dL (males) or > 1.8 mg/dL (females) should not be treated with eplerenone.[127]

SIDE EFFECTS

The major concern with eplerenone therapy is hyperkalemia. Potassium retention is a consequence of aldosterone blockade, and therefore careful monitoring of potassium levels is necessary. The risk of hyperkalemia is greater in patients with renal failure and with a history of diabetes. Since the hyperkalemia is affected by the dose of eplerenone, dose adjustment and careful monitoring of potassium and renal function are especially important in diabetic patients and patients with preexisting renal dysfunction.

Because eplerenone is metabolized through the cytochrome P450 3A4 system, it should not be used with inhibitors of that system such as ketoconazole, erythromycin, and verapamil.

USE OF THE ALDOSTERONE RECEPTOR BLOCKER

While eplerenone does have an FDA indication for the treatment of hypertension, the focus of its use should be in the management of severe heart failure, as additional therapy beyond ACE inhibitors and/or ARBs and beta-blockers, and in other therapy. I think its use in uncomplicated hypertension, with the profusion of other agents available, is not appropriate.

Chapter 11
Central Agonists

The central agonists work through the central nervous system (CNS). They include several of the older medications that were important for therapy at the beginning of the blood pressure control era in the 1970s. However, since they work in the CNS, they frequently have CNS side effects that limit, appropriately so, their use to unusual situations. Also, their 1 attractive feature in the last decade—low cost—has become moot as many of the very well-tolerated classes like the ACE inhibitors and CCBs have become generic.

MECHANISM OF ACTION

The central agonists bind at the alpha-2 receptor in the CNS. This binding stimulates the alpha-adrenergic system, resulting in decreased sympathetic outflow to the heart, kidneys, and the peripheral vessels. This reduced sympathetic outflow reduces cardiac output while relaxing the arterial tone, with both mechanisms lowering blood pressure.

EVIDENCE OF EFFICACY

No specific long-term events reduction trials show that treatment with these agents will reduce cardiovascular events along with controlling blood pressure. They were used several times as secondary agents in some of the early hypertension trials, but it is not possible to sort out any particular proof of efficacy from the data. Our experience with their blood pressure lowering shows that their hypertensive effect, at least initially, is equivalent to other monotherapy medications.

One of these agents, clonidine, has had beneficial CNS effects in the treatment of other conditions, including prophylaxis of vascular headache (migraine), reduction of systemic symptoms of opioid withdrawal, and management of dysmenorrheal syndromes.

AGENTS AND DOSAGE

There are 4 central alpha agonists currently on the US market. They share the mechanism of action, and they share similar CNS side effects (fatigue, depression, mental confusion, sedation, and dizziness) in addition to other agent-specific issues.

The agents and their traditional doses are listed in Table 11-1, along with some of their combination products.

SIDE EFFECTS

The considerable side effect pattern of these agents presented major problems for patient compliance in the 1970s when they were among the most commonly used agents. Therefore, when the ACE inhibitors and CCBs, with their very mild side effect profiles, emerged, the use of these agents fell dramatically.

All of the agents have *significant* CNS side effects, including sedation, fatigue, depression, dizziness, mental confusion, and dry mouth. These side effects are dose dependent, so that lower doses do have lower levels of these problems. The clonidine transdermal patch releases a lower level of clonidine over the week of its use, with some diminution of its CNS side effects, but many patients are not comfortable with wearing the patch for a full week.

Table 11-1 Central Alpha-2 Agonists

Agents	Usual Doses	Schedule
Clonidine (Catapres)	0.1–0.8 mg	Twice/day
Clonidine transdermal patch	0.1–0.2 mg	1/week
Guanabenz (Wytensin)	4–16 mg	Twice/day
Guanfacine (Tenex)	1–3 mg	Daily
Methyldopa (Aldomet)	250–1000 mg	Twice/day
Combination		
Clonidine/chlorthalidone	0.1/15 mg, 0.2/15 mg	Once or twice daily
Methyldopa/HCTZ	250/15 mg, 250/25 mg, 500/30 mg, 500/50 mg	Once or twice daily

The more agent-specific side effects are also an issue. Clonidine has 1 particular issue, which is the potential for a "rebound" adrenergic overdrive if it is stopped abruptly. Methyldopa has several specific side effects, including abnormal liver function tests, black tongue, and an autoimmune disorder with a positive Coombs' test and even hemolytic anemia.

USE OF THE CENTRAL AGONISTS

These agents have a limited usefulness in the management of hypertension. Because of the significant side effect profiles, they should only be used as supplemental agents in patients with very difficult-to-manage hypertension, often as an additional agent (in the lowest possible doses) in a patient on the full range of other medications.

Chapter 12
Direct Vasodilators

Two agents are available in this class, hydralazine and minoxidil. These agents are effective at lowering blood pressure, even in very difficult-to-treat patients. However, they do have significant side effect profiles that severely restrict their use to patients who are very difficult to manage. Hydralazine is also used in an intravenous infusion in severe hypertension situations, including preeclampsia of pregnancy. Minoxidil has, of course, enjoyed great success in a topical preparation for restoring or maintaining hair growth in men and women with hair loss. Hydralazine has recently been developed as a combination product with isosorbide dinitrate (BiDil) to treat severe heart failure in African American patients.

MECHANISM OF ACTION

The exact cellular mechanism whereby each of these agents lowers blood pressure is not clear. However, it appears that each agent (perhaps through different mechanisms) directly relaxes the smooth muscles around the arterial system, thus lowering the blood pressure. Since they appear to work directly at the arterial smooth muscle, without any other effect on the cardiac system, they frequently produce a reflex tachycardia, a significant increase in stroke volume, and an increase in cardiac output. They can also activate the RAAS, leading to sodium and water retention. Both of these actions, particularly the cardiac stimulation, can lead to new-onset angina and peripheral edema.

EVIDENCE OF EFFICACY

Hydralazine was used as a third-step agent in several of the early hypertension trials, but it is not possible to sort out its efficacy from that of the other primary agents used. The only clear efficacy trials for these agents are when hydralazine has been used in conjunction with isosorbide dinitrate for the treatment of heart failure. An early small study showed a reduction in cardiovascular mortality when the combination was utilized.[128] A much larger study in African American heart failure patients showed a major reduction in mortality and hospitalizations when added to comprehensive therapy.[129]

Outside of these heart failure studies, there are no long-term events reduction data for either hydralazine or minoxidil.

AGENTS AND DOSAGE

Hydralazine is dosed 2, 3, or 4 times a day, beginning at 40 mg/day (either 10 mg given 4 times per day or 20 mg twice daily). The dose is increased to 100 mg/day after 3 or more days, and then up to 200 mg/day (probably as 100 mg twice daily). Minoxidil is initially begun as an initial dose of 5 mg/day. It is then increased to 10 to 40 mg/day in either once- or twice-daily doses.

SIDE EFFECTS

The side effects of both of these agents are profound and severely limit their usefulness. Many of the side effects are the direct result of the actions of the agents with their direct vasodilatation without other cardiac mechanisms. The reflex increase in myocardial contractility and oxygen demand frequently leads to new-onset angina unless they are used in conjunction with a beta-blocker. Flushing is also commonly seen. The activation of the RAAS frequently leads to *severe* sodium and volume retention, frequently requiring aggressive loop diuretics like furosemide to control the edema.

Hydralazine frequently causes the appearance of positive ANA levels, and can even produce a lupus-like clinical syndrome. Minoxidil will increase hair growth diffusely.

USE OF THE DIRECT VASODILATORS

In the management of hypertension, these agents have a very limited role, since their side effects are so significant and difficult to manage. Hydralazine does have use in special roles, like intravenously in crises situations. It also has usefulness in the management of heart failure in its combination product (BiDil) in African Americans who require treatment beyond the ACE inhibitor, ARB, and beta-blocker regimens. Since this combination product is relatively new, its usefulness and impact in practice remain to be determined.

It is unlikely that many practitioners will need to resort to using these agents.

Chapter 13

Peripheral Adrenergic Inhibitors

There are 3 agents in this category. One of these agents, reserpine, had extensive use, both as a monotherapy agent and in combination preparations. One combination, marketed as Ser-Ap-Es, was a widely used low-dose combination of reserpine, hydralazine, and a thiazide. The other 2 agents are guanethidine and guanadrel, and they are potent agents that tend to be used uncommonly and in more difficult patients.

MECHANISM OF ACTION

These 3 agents share a similar, but not identical, mechanism. They block the effects of the sympathetic nervous system by transporting norepinephrine into the storage granules at the receptors and also by inhibiting their release. These effects are probably seen both peripherally and centrally and lead to the blood pressure lowering and the side effects.

The blood pressure lowering is similar to that seen with other hypertensive medications. The side effects, however, are considerable and have led to a near complete cessation of their use as the modern and better-tolerated agents became available.

The site of the action of these agents on the neurotransmitters often leads to significant CNS side effects (depression, sexual dysfunction, and dizziness). Also, both guanethidine and guanadrel have the potential for producing orthostatic hypotension, which can be significant.

Table 13-1 Peripheral Adrenergic Inhibitors

Agent	Usual Doses	Schedule
Guanadrel (Hylorel)	10–20 mg	2/day
Guanethidine (Ismelin)	10–20 mg	1/day
Reserpine	0.05–0.1 mg	1/day

EVIDENCE OF EFFICACY

Reserpine was used as a secondary agent in some of the early hypertension trials. However, we cannot separate out any specific effect that it may have had in the overall trial.

AGENTS AND DOSAGE

The agents and their traditional doses are listed in Table 13-1.

SIDE EFFECTS

As previously stated, the significant side effect pattern of these agents has severely limited their use. The side effects are predominantly CNS-related (depression, sexual dysfunction, and dizziness), and there is also the potential for orthostatic hypotension with some of the agents.

USE OF THE PERIPHERAL ADRENERGIC INHIBITORS

These agents currently have a very limited use, since their side effects make them much less attractive than the more modern agents. There are some physicians who support the use of reserpine in low doses, where the side effects are reduced, but this is not common at this time. Therefore, I think the peripheral adrenergic inhibitors will remain agents with quite limited use in the modern era.

Section 2

Cholesterol

Chapter 14
Hyperlipidemia

Elevated cholesterol has long been associated with an increased risk for coronary artery disease, along with other forms of atherosclerosis. The original information was based on observational, population-based studies. In these studies, populations with generally higher cholesterol levels, like those in the United States in the 1950s and 1960s, were found to have significantly higher rates of coronary disease than populations with very low cholesterol levels, like certain East Asian or African populations. Our much higher cholesterol diet here in the United States was implicated as a major causative factor in this problem, as evidenced by the discovery that within 2 generations of arriving in the United States, immigrant groups from lower heart disease areas, like East Asia, would see their cholesterol and their risk for coronary heart disease (CHD) climb toward the level of other US populations.

Observing these facts, there was a slowly progressing national interest in reducing the cholesterol content of our diet, with the appearance of many "low fat" and "lite" foods, along with a move away from "red meat" to poultry and fish. Whether these dietary changes had a significantly positive impact is not the focus of this book.

As interest in the cholesterol question emerged several decades ago, our therapeutic options were hampered by limited therapeutic data. The early cholesterol medication trials were only modestly successful, and that led some scientists and lay observers to challenge the "cholesterol hypothesis," the belief that reducing cholesterol would lead to a reduction in coronary artery and other atherosclerotic diseases.

The original US cholesterol therapy trial was the Coronary Drug Project, which evaluated several different therapies in men with known CHD. Clofibrate (the original marketed fibrate agent) and high-dose niacin (3.0 grams daily) showed no reduction in total or cardiac mortality over the 5 years of the study in these high-risk men.[130] There was a reduction in nonfatal MI in the niacin group, but this was in a secondary endpoint only.[130] Another large clofibrate trial in Europe showed a reduction in nonfatal MI, but no reduction in fatal MI, and an *increase* in total mortality with clofibrate.[131]

The only significant trial with a resin binding agent was the LRC-CPPT trial, which used 24 gm/day of cholestyramine resin in men with elevated cholesterol but without known heart disease ("primary prevention"). After 7.4 years, the resin-treated patients had a significant reduction (19%) in fatal or nonfatal MI.[132] The final early study was the Helsinki Heart Study, a primary prevention trial in Finland. The gemfibrozil-treated patients, as compared to the placebo-treated patients, also had a reduction in MI, but they also did not have a reduction in total or cardiac mortality.[133] These results, in summary, were suggestive but not overwhelming in their support of cholesterol modification by medication to prevent heart disease. The overwhelming evidence was to come later, with the trials of "statins," as HMG-CoA reductase inhibitors have come to be called.

The first NIH recommendation directed at the importance of lowering cholesterol to reduce the risk of CHD was not until 1985.[134] This recommendation was not universally accepted by all interested groups, with often quite public challenges to the "cholesterol hypothesis" by certain individuals.

This confusion was more related to the modest benefit of the agents that were available for the original trials, including fibrate products like gemfibrozil and clofibrate, along with the resin binders like cholestyramine. These agents had modest cholesterol reduction benefits that led to modest events reductions or events reductions that were mainly in certain subgroups. Only when the HMG-CoA reductase inhibitors (statins) came into use with their dramatic cholesterol reduction potency did the science become very clear about the power of cholesterol reduction with those agents to reduce cardiac events.

EPIDEMIOLOGY AND IMPACT

The landmark Framingham Heart Study that began in Massachusetts in the 1940s found that the risk of developing CHD in the lifetime of a 40-year-old is 1 in 2 for men and 1 in 3 for women.[135] This considerable risk demands that we make every reasonable effort to determine the causes of this epidemic, then treat whatever causes we can to slow this widespread and common disease.

Over the last several decades, a clear consensus has emerged that elevated cholesterol, particularly elevated low-density lipoprotein cholesterol (LDL-C) is a clear and direct cause of atherosclerosis and its manifestations, especially presenting as coronary artery disease. The clearest statement of this is in the Third Report of the National Cholesterol Education Panel (ATP-III), issued in 2001 and updated in 2004. In this 2001 report, the expert panel summarized the data, concluding that both the epidemiological and treatment data pointed to elevated LDL-C as the *principal* (but not only) risk factor for CHD, and therefore the principal treatment target for cholesterol therapy.[136]

The report drew heavily on earlier epidemiological studies that documented the relationship between cholesterol abnormalities and the risk of CHD. Analysis from the MRFIT study in 1986 clearly demonstrated that elevated cholesterol increased the risk for CHD in a continuous and graded fashion, meaning that the risk continued to increase as the cholesterol increased.[137] At the same time, the landmark Framingham Heart Study showed that low HDL-C (high-density lipoprotein cholesterol) and elevated total cholesterol also increased the risk for CHD progressively throughout middle age.[138] Subsequent data from Framingham showed the increased CHD risk from elevated cholesterol extended to include older-age patients, not just the middle-aged patients who had been included in the earlier studies.[139]

Other reports from Framingham added further support to the importance of cardiac risks from elevated cholesterol. These follow-up manuscripts documented that the risk was present in patients with previous heart disease ("secondary prevention") and in patients without previous heart disease ("primary prevention").[140–142] Similar data from other study groups also confirmed the importance of cholesterol elevation leading to CHD.[143–145] Finally, the Framingham database was used to calculate a 10-year risk algorithm for the development of CHD, based on age, gender, blood pressure, smoking, HDL-C, and total cholesterol.[146] This algorithm was adopted by the ATP-III panel to be used nationally for screening disease-free patients for their risk of developing CHD over the next 10 years.

Finally, the strongest evidence for the importance of managing elevated cholesterol in the prevention of CHD has been the dramatic reduction in cardiac disease mortality noted over the last 30 years. This reduction has been closely associated with a significant reduction in serum cholesterol values between 1960 and 2002, a reduction due to the expanding use of aggressive lipid lowering medications.[147] While many people stress dietary management of cholesterol, US evidence shows that dietary counseling programs have no impact on the risk of CHD, stroke, or cardiovascular disease.[148] This very clear and powerful message is that the way to attack cholesterol is with aggressive medication therapy.

Chapter 15

Diagnosis and Risk Stratification

The diagnostic and risk stratification guidelines for cholesterol management were summarized in the ATP-III report in 2001 and updated in a follow-up report in 2004.[136,149]

The reports stratified risk for MI in the next 10 years from the Framingham Heart Study. In the 2001 report, they defined 3 classifications of potential risk: CHD or CHD risk equivalents, 2 or more risk factors, or 0 to 1 risk factors. These risk factors are listed in Table 15-1 and include the following:

- Cigarette smoking
- Hypertension (either an elevated blood pressure or on antihypertensive medication)
- Low HDL-C (< 40 mg/dL)
- A family history of premature heart disease (defined as CHD developing in a first-degree male relative < 55 years or a first-degree female relative < 65 years)
- Age (males ≥ 45 years; females ≥ 55 years)

Simply count up the potential 5 risk factors, allowing for a subtraction of 1 if the patient has an HDL ≥ 60.

Then consult the risk calculation table (Table 15-2), which predicts the risk of an MI over the next 10 years:

Table 15-1 Major Risk Factors for CHD

Cigarette smoking
Hypertension, either a blood pressure of ≥ 140/90 mm Hg or treatment with antihypertensive medication
Low HDL cholesterol (< 40 mg/dL)
Family history of premature coronary heart disease, in a first-degree male relative < 55 years or female relative < 65 years
Age ≥ 45 years for men and ≥ 55 years for women

Table 15-2 Risk of Myocardial Infarction Over the Next 10 Years

Age Points			
Men		Women	
Age	Points	Age	Points
20–34	−9	20–34	−7
35–39	−4	35–39	−3
40–44	0	40–44	0
45–49	3	45–49	3
50–54	6	50–54	6
55–59	8	55–59	8
60–64	10	60–64	10
65–69	11	65–69	12
70–74	12	70–74	14
75–79	13	75–79	16

Total Cholesterol Points										
	Age									
	Men					Women				
	20–39	40–49	50–59	60–69	70–79	20–39	40–49	50–59	60–69	70–79
< 160	0	0	0	0	0	0	0	0	0	0
160–199	4	3	2	1	0	4	3	2	1	1
200–239	7	5	3	1	0	8	6	4	2	1
240–279	9	6	4	2	1	11	8	5	3	2
≥ 280	11	8	5	3	1	13	10	7	4	2

Table 15-2 Risk of Myocardial Infarction Over the Next 10 Years (cont'd)

Smoking Points										
	Age									
	Men					Women				
	20–39	40–49	50–59	60–69	70–79	20–39	40–49	50–59	60–69	70–79
Nonsmoker	0	0	0	0	0	0	0	0	0	0
Smoker	8	5	3	1	1	9	7	4	2	1

Low HDL-C Points			
Men		Women	
HDL, mg/dL	Points	HDL, mg/dL	Points
≥ 60	−1	≥ 60	−1
50–59	0	50–59	0
40–49	1	40–49	1
< 40	2	< 40	2

Blood Pressure Points					
Men			Women		
Systolic BP	If Untreated	Treated	Systolic BP	If Untreated	Treated
< 120	0	0	< 120	0	0
120–129	0	1	120–129	1	3
130–139	1	2	130–139	2	4
140–159	1	2	140–159	3	5
≥ 160	2	3	≥ 160	4	6

Table 15-2 Risk of Myocardial Infarction Over the Next 10 Years (cont'd)

Total Risk			
Men		Women	
Points	10-Year Risk, %	Points	10-Year Risk, %
< 0	< 1	< 9	< 1
0	1	9	1
1	1	10	1
2	1	11	1
3	1	12	1
4	1	13	2
5	2	14	2
6	2	15	3
7	3	16	4
8	4	17	5
9	5	18	6
10	6	19	8
11	8	20	11
12	10	21	14
13	12	22	17
14	16	23	22
15	20	24	27
16	25	≥ 25	≥ 30

A quick glance shows the well-known difference in risk for MI, at least at earlier ages, between men and women. While as many women as men have MIs over their lifetime, men develop them at a much earlier age.

This difference shows up clearly in the risk scales. To get to the moderate risk level, say 10% over the next 10 years, a man needs only 12 points, while a woman needs 20. If all of the parameters are equal, such as blood pressure and cholesterol values, a woman would be about 10 years older than a man to be at the same degree of risk of an MI.

It is important to recognize that many patients who appear to be low risk in routine practice, say a 55-year-old nonsmoking man with hypertension controlled to a systolic blood pressure of 132 mm Hg and what appears to be borderline cholesterol (total cholesterol of 210 mg/dL and

HDL-C of 44 mg/dL) would actually fall into the moderate risk group (age 55 = 8 points; treated systolic blood pressure of 132 mm Hg = 2 points; total cholesterol 210 mg/dL = 3 points; HDL-C 44 mg/dL = 1 point). These 14 points add up to a 16% risk of MI in the next 10 years. Therefore, it is critical that all middle-aged patients, particularly those with hypertension, even if it is well controlled, should have their cholesterol carefully screened. Computing the risk from this table takes only seconds, and it can be crucial for the well-being of many of your patients.

The diagnostic and treatment target is the LDL-C. Although the LDL-C is not used to *calculate* the risk, it is the treatment target for cholesterol management. While there is concern about other lipid fractions, like HDL-C and triglycerides, and subfractions, there is clear consensus that, at this time, the LDL-C remains the treatment target.[149] Proper measurement of the LDL-C is obtained through a fasting lipid panel, including the total cholesterol, LDL-C, HDL-C, and triglycerides. This panel requires a 12-hour fast, usually overnight, with no calories consumed during the 12 hours. The fast is necessary to obtain an accurate triglyceride measurement, which is used to calculate the LDL-C (LDL-C = total-C – HDL-C – [triglycerides/5]). Some research trials are now using a direct LDL-C measurement, but in general it is too cumbersome and expensive for routine clinical use. The calculated LDL-C, which was used in many of the early treatment trials, is sufficient for routine use. While some research projects use an average of 2 lipid values, in clinical practice we frequently use a single lipid panel to assess whether to institute treatment with a cholesterol lowering agent.

While many clinicians consider that the other lipid fractions, including low HDL-C or elevated triglycerides, may deserve treatment, there is not a consensus about these fractions, including whether they should be treated, and especially how they should be treated, and finally what the treatment targets for low HDL-C or elevated triglycerides might be. This lack of clarity may be answered in the future by ongoing research trials, but until they might be completed, lowering of elevated LDL-C remains our only clear and definitive treatment target.

Chapter 16

Treatment Issues

TREATMENT TARGETS FOR LDL-C

The treatment targets and goals for LDL-C are based on the presence of preexisting atherosclerotic disease or on the risk for atherosclerotic disease of the individual, as measured by the Framingham risk scale discussed in Chapter 15. I will present the targets/goals based on the risk group for the patient.

Please note that the *high-risk group* includes many millions of patients, often those patients who you do not suspect as being high risk. This group includes all patients with any of the following conditions:

- Any form of coronary artery disease, including patients with a recent or remote diagnosis of acute MI, angina pectoris, coronary angioplasty or bypass grafting, or a history of acute coronary syndrome
- Cerebrovascular disease, including all patients with recent or remote cerebrovascular accident or transient ischemic attack
- Peripheral artery disease, including those with symptomatic or asymptomatic claudication
- Diabetes mellitus
- Global risk calculation of > 20% or more, a category that will include most hypertensive men above 65 years and most hypertensive women above 75 years

The *moderately high-risk* group also includes many millions of patients, again many more than you might at first suspect. This group has 2 or more risk factors, such as a male above

45 years (one factor) with an HDL-C < 40 (a second factor), or a 55-year-old female (one factor) with hypertension (a second factor). This group has a calculated 10-year risk of 10% to 20%. The *moderate-risk group* is also defined by 2 or more risk factors, but with a calculated risk of < 10%.

Finally, the *low-risk group* has 0 to 1 risk factor, and these individuals almost always have a global risk of < 10%, so that the calculation of the 10-year risk is not recommended. Only small numbers of individuals with very high cholesterol in this group will need treatment.[150] (See Table 16-1.)

In the future, the LDL-C targets listed previously may continue to drop to lower levels. Early research trials have begun to point to lower targets, both in patients with CHD and in lower-risk patients. The newer studies have used imaging techniques to monitor the extent of atherosclerotic plaque burden in the carotid or coronary arteries. After aggressive cholesterol lowering treatment, the measurements were repeated to evaluate plaque progression, stabilization, or regression. One trial in low-risk patients, METEOR, lowered the LDL-C to 78 mg/dL and achieved plaque stabilization in the carotid arteries on ultrasound.[150] Two other studies in high-risk individuals lowered the LDL-C to 79 mg/dL or 72 mg/dL, producing plaque stabilization or slight plaque regression.[151,152] Also, a rosuvastatin trial, ASTEROID, was able to lower LDL-C to 61 mg/dL and achieve a modest (9%), but definite, degree of plaque regression.[153]

Finally, the recently published JUPITER trial provides solid evidence for considering lower LDL-C target levels in patients without previous cardiovascular disease. In JUPITER, patients with LDL-C < 130 mg/dL but with an elevated hs-CRP (high-sensitivity C-reactive protein) inflammation marker were randomized to rosuvastatin (20 mg) or placebo. The LDL-C in the rosuvastatin-treated group dropped to 55 mg/dL, and there were massive reductions in cardiovascular events. The combined endpoint was reduced by 44%, nonfatal MI was reduced by 65%, total MI was reduced by 54%, and even total mortality was reduced by 20%. These event reductions were about twice what was expected at the beginning of the study.[154]

There will probably be vigorous debate over the significance of this study. Many people will reemphasize the utilization of hs-CRP in screening. I think the greatest significance is in the LDL-C levels achieved. This is the first study to treat at-risk patients down to LDL-C levels in the 55 mg/dL range. What it may indicate is that, with our current guidelines, we may be undertreating everyone. Whether this type of data will lead to further reductions in LDL-C targets is unclear, but it certainly makes a strong argument in favor of significantly lower LDL-C treatment targets in the future.

Table 16-1 Risk for Atherosclerotic Disease

Risk Category	LDL-C Goal	Consider Drug Therapy
High Risk	< 100 mg/dL < 70 mg/dL optional goal[a]	≥ 100 mg/dL < 100 mg/dL
Moderately High Risk 2+ risk factors with 10%–20% 10-year risk	< 130 mg/dL < 100 mg/dL optional goal[a]	≥ 130 mg/dL 100–129 mg/dL

Table 16-1 Risk for Atherosclerotic Disease Cont'd

Risk Category	LDL-C Goal	Consider Drug Therapy
Moderate Risk 2+ risk factors with < 10% ten-year risk	< 130 mg/dL	≥ 160 mg/dL
Lower Risk 0–1 risk factors	< 160 mg/dL	≥ 190 mg/dL 160–189 mg/dL

[a]Noted optional targets are recommended as preferred targets by this author.

OTHER LIPID FRACTIONS

Two other lipid fractions have generated considerable interest, and some controversy, about whether, and especially how, they should be treated. These are, of course, triglycerides and HDL-C. While the importance of diagnosing and treating LDL-C has been established and confirmed many times, there is a significant lack of confirming evidence for the other 2 lipid fractions.

Low HDL-C has long been recognized as a potent risk factor for the development of atherosclerotic cardiovascular disease. Low HDL-C is currently defined as < 40mg/dL, both in men and women.[136] The increased risk from low HDL-C has been extensively documented in many studies, and it is a relatively common finding, seen in about one-third of adult males and one-fifth of adult women. Low HDL-C is frequently seen in combination with elevated triglycerides, abdominal obesity, and insulin resistance in the metabolic syndrome. The increased cardiovascular risk from low HDL-C extends across all age groups, even into the elderly.[155] Also, secondary analyses from several trials that treated elevated LDL-C with aggressive statin therapy found that the risk caused by low HDL-C was persistent even with aggressive statin therapy.[156,157]

However, treatment questions around low HDL-C are very difficult. The ATP-III panel does not make any specific recommendations as to when or even how treatment for low HDL-C should be undertaken. A careful look at the available data will show how difficult the treatment question for low HDL-C is.

Practitioners who advocate for treating low HDL-C point to 2 older studies utilizing gemfibrozil, a fibric acid agent that raises HDL-C and lowers triglycerides, as support for treatment to raise HDL-C. However, both of the studies were completed in the era *before* the statins (HMG-CoA reductase inhibitors) came onto the market. Therefore, they do *not* offer any information about whether combining a fibric acid agent, like fenofibrate, might further reduce cardiovascular events greater than just using a statin alone as monotherapy. Indeed, gemfibrozil, in my opinion, should *never* be combined with a statin, since gemfibrozil interferes with the glucuronidation metabolism of the statins, leading to potentially toxic levels of statin.[158]

The Helsinki Heart Study, a trial in high-risk individuals without known heart disease, studied gemfibrozil versus placebo. The results showed a modest but significant reduction in initial

MI in the gemfibrozil-treated patients but did not show a reduction in total or cardiovascular mortality.[133] A follow-up analysis attributed the events reduction with gemfibrozil to the increases in HDL-C and also to LDL-C lowering from the gemfibrozil but not to the reduction in triglycerides that also occurred.[159] The VA HIT trial was a US trial utilizing gemfibrozil versus placebo in patients with coronary disease ("secondary patients") with HDL-C < 40 mg/dL and LDL-C about 111 mg/dL.[160] In this study, gemfibrozil treatment resulted in a 22% reduction in nonfatal MI, attributed in a subsequent evaluation to the 6% increase in HDL-C but not to the triglyceride reduction.[161]

While niacin, or nicotinic acid, therapy does increase HDL-C, whether this HDL-C effect will result in cardiac events reduction has never been proven.

The most definitive study on how to treat patients with low HDL-C syndrome, at least in primary preventive patients, is the AFCAPS/TexCAPS study. This primary prevention study identified men and women with mid-range LDL-C elevation (mean 150 mg/dL) and with low HDL-C of 36 mg/dL in men and 40mg/dL in women. Treatment with lovastatin versus placebo significantly reduced first cardiovascular events throughout the study.[162] Interestingly, in the patients with HDL-C of < 40 mg/dL, the events reduction was dramatic, with an events reduction of just less than 50%.[163] This could be attributed to the 25% reduction in LDL-C or the 6% increase in HDL-C, or the combination. However, it does provide us with an easy and well-proven way to treat low HDL-C, namely by utilizing aggressive statin therapy.

The difficult HDL-C question is further complicated by secondary analyses of 2 cholesterol studies, IDEAL and EPIC, which seemed to imply that high plasma HDL-C and large HDL particle size *increase*, not decrease, cardiac risk—a strikingly unexpected finding.[164] Finally, the Torcetrapib story also clouds the HDL-C picture. Torcetrapib was a CETP inhibitor that produced a dramatic 72% increase in HDL-C along with a 25% reduction in LDL-C. It was to be paired with atorvastatin by its manufacturer, and it had enormous potential to dominate the cholesterol market in the future. However, torcetrapib produced an increase in cardiac mortality and MI.[165] The mechanisms for this absence of benefit coupled with the dramatic cardiovascular toxicity are unclear and may never be resolved.

Therefore, at this point, the clearest and most proven way to treat low HDL-C syndrome is with aggressive statin therapy, as in the AFCAPS/TexCAPS study. There are studies underway assessing combination therapy with a statin combined with niacin or a statin combined with fenofibrate (versus statin therapy alone), to evaluate whether these additional treatments to raise HDL-C or lower triglycerides will reduce events further than statin therapy alone. Whether these research studies will resolve our question is unclear for at least the near future. It is possible that HDL-C will remain a marker of increased cardiac risk without clear evidence that treating it will be beneficial.[166]

TRIGLYCERIDES

The question of triglycerides remains one of the more confusing issues in the management of lipid disorders. Having been on the national lecture circuit for many years, I have seen more confusion around this issue than any other in cholesterol management.

First, we need to clarify a diagnostic matter. There are many types of triglyceride disorders, with varying degrees of frequency and disease impact. In the old Frederickson classification system, the cholesterol disorders we see frequently in clinical practice and treat to reduce early CHD are type II-A, where LDL-C is significantly elevated and HDL-C and triglycerides are relatively normal, and type II-B, where LDL-C is elevated, HDL-C is decreased, and triglycerides are increased. Type II-B is frequently seen in the metabolic syndrome. These 2 disorders are common and require aggressive management.

There is a less common but still noticeable disorder, type IV in the Frederickson classification system. This disorder is seen once in every 500 individuals and represents a different genetic disorder. It is characterized by significant triglyceride elevation of > 500 mg/dL, normal total cholesterol (< 250 mg/dL), normal or low LDL-C, and low HDL-C. This disorder is not associated with an increased risk for coronary or other atherosclerotic disease, so statin treatment is not indicated. It is associated with pancreatitis. Initial treatment is best managed through lifestyle issues, combining an exercise program with a low-fat, low-carbohydrate diet. Medication treatment would be with a fibrate, if medication was felt to be indicated. It is not clear if medication treatment will avoid future bouts of pancreatitis. If pancreatitis does occur in this disorder, an aggressive investigation for gallstones is very important.

However, triglyceride elevation is much more commonly seen as another component in the complex cholesterol disorder along with an elevated LDL-C and a low HDL-C (type II-B disease), which is the cholesterol picture frequently seen in metabolic syndrome and diabetes mellitus. This cholesterol pattern is frequently associated with an increased risk for coronary and other atherosclerosis, leading many authors and indeed the ATP-III panel to recommend *considering* treating elevated triglycerides along with the elevated LDL-C.

The emphasis I added in the previous sentence is important, since the ATP-III panel recommended only "considering" treatment of patients with elevated triglycerides when they are in the 200 through 499 mg/dL range.[136] They do not, however, offer specific treatment initiation thresholds to start therapy, nor do they offer specific triglyceride treatment target levels for reduction. This hesitancy on the part of the ATP-III panel is appropriate, considering there is no clinical trial evidence to support such a recommendation or to identify triglyceride levels at which to begin treatment or triglyceride levels to be the targets for treatment.

Since many practitioners are not aware of this ambivalence on the part of the ATP-III panel, I think that a careful review of the science is appropriate in considering whether we should recommend treatment of triglycerides or not. When traditional studies look at triglyceride elevations as isolated factors, and not as part of an overall pattern of lipid abnormalities that includes low HDL-C and other factors, they clearly find an *association* between elevated triglycerides and CHD.[167] However, when other studies examine the complex mix of other coronary disease risk factors in patients with elevated triglycerides, they find that the elevation of risk from the triglycerides becomes much less, often fading to borderline significance or even disappearing.[168,169] It appears that low HDL-C levels, which are frequently seen with elevated triglycerides, may account for much of the presumed triglyceride risk.[170] Therefore, elevated triglycerides may mainly be a *marker*, or surrogate, for the complex of cardiac risk factors like low HDL-C rather than an independent risk factor.

Firm conclusions are difficult to gather from the few treatment trials that have evaluated the impact of treatment on triglycerides and cardiac events. The fundamental problem in examining these trials is that they were not designed to determine whether lowering triglycerides reduced cardiac events. Rather, they evaluated the effects of certain cholesterol medications, statins and fibrates, on reducing cardiac events. After the studies were completed, secondary analyses of the data included evaluations of the effects of triglyceride levels or triglyceride lowering on events. Since these evaluations are the secondary rather than the primary intent of the studies, they are *suggestive* rather than *definitive*.

Two large trials used gemfibrozil, a fibrate agent, to reduce cardiac events in patients without and with previous coronary disease, the Helsinki Heart Study and the VA HIT study. Both studies showed that gemfibrozil reduced cardiac events, but analyses of the data showed that this reduction was not significantly associated with a reduction in triglycerides, but rather was due to effects principally on HDL-C.[159,161] Similar post-hoc evaluations have looked at triglyceride effects in several of the statin trials. In 2 of the original statin trials, West of Scotland and 4S, follow-up analyses found that the risk of elevated triglycerides disappeared in the groups on statin therapy, especially when HDL-C was factored in.[171,172] An analysis of the IDEAL study found a similar effect, where on treatment, triglycerides did not affect cardiac event rates when the HDL-C was factored in.[173] Only 1 statin trial, the PROVE-IT TIMI 22 trial, which compared 2 different statins, found that lower triglycerides were associated with lower events.[174] However, since the 2 studied statins, atorvastatin and pravastatin, had dramatically different effects on triglycerides, LDL-C, and other factors, this different result may primarily be due to the different agents used.

In summary, there certainly is no clear information about medication treatment of elevated triglycerides: whether lowering them with medication will reduce cardiac events, what levels of elevated triglycerides warrant treatment and what our targets levels for treatment should be, or what agents should be used and at what doses. With all this uncertainty, I do not recommend adding a second agent to reduce moderately elevated triglycerides. In high-cholesterol patients, I aggressively lower their LDL-C with statin therapy, then try to lower any residual triglyceride elevation with an exercise program and a low-fat, low-carbohydrate diet. The lifestyle approach is especially important in metabolic syndrome patients, where the potential for the development of diabetes mellitus is extremely high. In these patients, lifestyle management to avoid the evolution from metabolic syndrome to frank diabetes mellitus is critical.

NON–HIGH-DENSITY LIPOPROTEIN CHOLESTEROL

In the ATP-III report, rather than recommend specific treatment for elevated triglycerides, where there is no specific research data to guide us in how we should implement or proceed with such treatment, the panel advocated the calculation of non–HDL-C in patients with triglycerides > 200 mg/dL as a *secondary calculation*. The non–HDL-C is calculated by subtracting the HDL-C from the total cholesterol (TC–HDL-C = non–HDL-C). This calculation is designed to incorporate the very low-density lipoprotein (VLDL), which carries remnant cholesterol, into a combination with the LDL-C. The normal/target values for the non–HDL-C are 30 mg/dL *greater* than the LDL-C normal/target values.

Some authors calculate that the non–HDL-C is a more accurate predictor of cardiac mortality than the LDL-C.[175] Other authors dispute that claim, asserting the value of non–HDL-C is not clear, since it incorporates the triglyceride value, with its uncertain impact, into the risk calculation.[176] Nevertheless, calculating the non–HDL-C, since it is recommended in the ATP-III report, is an acceptable way of incorporating elevated triglycerides into the risk calculation as a secondary calculation. Since this is a *secondary* calculation, its use may help if you desire another treatment target beyond using only the LDL-C. However, this is certainly an optional, not a mandatory, treatment target, and how often it is used in clinical practice is not known.

Whether this secondary calculation has any value in clinical practice is unclear, particularly since the treatment for elevated non–HDL-C is the same as the treatment for elevated LDL-C, namely aggressive statin therapy. In general, the use of aggressive statin therapy to lower LDL-C probably makes the calculation of non–HDL-C a minor issue for the busy practitioner.

LIPID SUBFRACTIONS

There are many subfractions of the various cholesterol components that are of considerable academic interest. Whether and how these emerging subfractions can or should be incorporated into clinical practice will not be clear for some time into the future.

The various subfractions include apolipoprotein B, which is the major atherogenic component of LDL-C; apolipoproteins A-I and A-II, which are components of HDL-C; lipoprotein (a), usually called Lp(a), which is a combination of LDL-C and a glycoprotein; and other subfractions, including apolipoprotein C and E, along with small dense LDL-C.

Current research has led several authors to conclude that certain subfractions may be better predictors of cardiovascular disease than the traditional components like LDL-C and HDL-C. Specifically, some authors assert that apolipoprotein B is a better predictor of cardiovascular events than is LDL-C, while others dispute that assertion.[177–181] Other interest focuses on the apolipoprotein B to apolipoprotein A-1 ratio as a superior predictor of events.[177]

At this stage of our knowledge, these questions remain very interesting but are outside of our treatment options. Even if the assertions about superior prediction of events by these subfractions are true, extensive clinical trials would have to be conducted to prove these assertions and to clearly define agents for treatment of events as well as guidelines and targets. These developments are in the distant future. We need to be open-minded about new and evolving information, but the subfraction question is still very preliminary and unclear.

Based on our current knowledge, the subfractions do not offer appropriate treatment issues for current clinical practice.

Chapter 17
Other Diagnostic Modalities

NON-LIPID MARKERS

There has been considerable research on other, non-lipid blood elements that might help indicate patients who are at increased risk of cardiovascular events. We always need to be cautious to avoid over-interpreting these markers. Remember that many studies showed an "association" between elevated levels of homocysteine and cardiovascular risk. However, many follow-up studies showed that treatment with folic acid would reduce the homocysteine to normal but would have no effect at all on the rate of cardiovascular events. Therefore, measuring homocysteine offers no therapeutic advantage in preventing cardiovascular events.[182]

The most prominent of the non-lipid blood markers currently is CRP, or C-reactive protein. Interest in CRP is as a marker for systemic inflammation, and the explanation for its usefulness in predicting cardiovascular events is that systemic inflammation predisposes atherosclerotic plaques to rupture, leading to acute occlusive events like MI. The CRP monitored in that context is a high-specificity CRP, a specific commercial test now widely available. The supporters of measuring and utilizing the CRP test in evaluating cardiovascular risk argue that the elevated CRP will indicate increased levels of systemic inflammation and that the inflammation will leave atherosclerotic plaques more vulnerable to plaque rupture leading to cardiovascular events like MI and stroke.

The evidence for measuring CRP originally came from Dr. Ridker's group, whose epidemiological studies showed the correlation between CRP elevation and cardiovascular risk.[183] Subsequently, other groups also showed a correlation in their epidemiological studies of elevated CRP and increased cardiovascular risk.[184–187]

Several other researchers, using similar epidemiological studies, did not find that the CRP correlation to increased cardiovascular risk was significant, leading many to question the importance of CRP measurement.[188–190] See Table 17-1 for a listing of CRP values and the risk elevation.

Further information from Dr. Ridker shows a correlation of elevated CRP with metabolic syndrome.[191–192] Some authors contend that the elevated CRP is not the cause of the inflammation, but simply an indicator, or marker, that it exists.[193–195] While some authors argue that routine CRP testing should be added to lipid screening, the Americana Heart Association (AHA) has been more cautious.[196]

In 2003, a position paper from the AHA noted that, in general, a significant elevation in CRP, to > 3.0 mg/L at most led to a doubling of cardiovascular risk calculation from the Framingham model.[196] Therefore, they recommended a limited utilization of the test to situations where a doubling of risk would change a person's prognosis and therefore treatment. Specifically, if a person's risk was in the 10% to 20% range, a CRP test would be useful, since a doubling of that risk would put the person into the high-risk category of > 20%. This remains a reasonable approach.

Ridker was able to identify a number of lifestyle and medication therapies that will reduce an elevated CRP.[197] (See Table 17-2) It is clear that many of these treatments listed in Table 17-2 will reduce cardiovascular risk while lowering CRP, including statins, exercise, and aspirin. Whether the CRP reduction causes the risk reduction or simply signifies it passively remains unclear.

The JUPITER study utilized an elevated CRP of > 2.0 mg/L to qualify patients for statin treatment even though their LDL was, at worst, borderline at < 130 mg/dL.[154] The dramatic reduction in all types of cardiovascular events and total mortality could be interpreted as support for more widespread use of the CRP test in screening moderate-risk individuals. The study could, in contrast, be interpreted simply as a mandate to be much more aggressive with the institution of statin therapy, including the treatment of low- and moderate-risk individuals with aggressive LDL lowering.

At this point, I think the AHA recommendation remains valid, that the real benefit of measuring CRP is confined to patients with moderate risk, in those with a global risk in the 10% to 20% range, where an elevated CRP should mandate aggressive statin therapy. In high-risk individuals, or in individuals where you intend to use aggressive statin therapy without the, CRP result, the test will not be helpful, since they already qualify for the appropriate therapy including statins, aspirin, weight management, and exercise. Also, in low-risk individuals, where the potential of doubling of cardiovascular risk would not necessitate statin treatment, say a person with a 2% risk that would double only to 4%, the test would be of no value.

Table 17-1 CRP (C-Reactive Protein) Values and Risk Elevation

CRP < 1.0 mg/L	Low risk with no risk elevation
CRP 1.0–3.0 mg/L	Intermediate risk with unclear effect on risk elevation
CRP > 3.0 mg/L	Increased risk, with the cardiovascular event risk increased by 50%–100%

Table 17-2 Factors That Reduce Elevated CRP

Aggressive statin therapy with LDL lowering
Aspirin
Diet, exercise, and weight loss
Smoking cessation

METABOLIC SYNDROME

Metabolic syndrome is the object of considerable interest, along with some confusion. It is not really a disease entity in itself, so we should not be diagnosing patients with it, even if they have it. It is, rather, a constellation of metabolic risk factors.[198] The syndrome does significantly predispose individuals with it to the development of diabetes, with about a 5-fold increase in diabetes (along with a doubling of the risk of cardiovascular disease). Unfortunately, there are several different definitions of metabolic syndrome, with some of the non-US ones requiring diabetes to be present.

Currently, most people in the United States use the definition presented in Table 17-3.[198] As you examine the table, you will quickly see that the syndrome is quite common, since we frequently find overweight patients with hypertension and low HDL-C or elevated triglycerides. On most occasions, we can quickly determine its presence by a quick look at the patient and the chart.

The presence of metabolic syndrome in itself does not add to the patient's cardiovascular risk. That risk is already somewhat advanced because of the presence of the multiple risk factors necessary to meet the criteria for the metabolic syndrome, so you would calculate the patient's risk from the Framingham risk calculation as in any other patient without metabolic syndrome.[198,199]

My own opinion is that the significance of determining the presence of the metabolic syndrome in a patient is that it signifies that the patient is at a very high risk of developing diabetes mellitus. Therefore, metabolic syndrome patients need to adopt aggressive lifestyle modification measures that will control this risk: exercise, diet and weight loss, and smoking cessation. There is no medication treatment for this situation, so lifestyle adjustment is critical.

ELECTRON-BEAM COMPUTERIZED TOMOGRAPHY OF THE HEART

The "heart scan," as it is commonly called, is an electron-beam computerized tomography (EBCT) scan of the heart that calculates the coronary artery calcification score in an effort to predict the extent of and risk for coronary artery disease with this noninvasive CT scan procedure. It is a popular and widely used test, but there is controversy as to how useful it really is in predicting and/or treating potential coronary artery disease.

Table 17-3 Criteria for Metabolic Syndrome (Meeting 3 of 5 Criteria Indicates Metabolic Syndrome)

Criteria	Measurement
Elevated Waist Circumference	≥ 102 cm in men ≥ 88 cm in women
Elevated Triglycerides (TG)	≥ 150 mg/dL or on treatment for elevated TG
Reduced HDL-C	< 40 mg/dL in men < 50 mg/dL in women, or on treatment for low HDL/C
Elevated Blood Pressure	≥ 130 mm Hg systolic BP or ≥ 85 mm Hg diastolic BP
Elevated Fasting Glucose	≥ 100 mg/dL or on treatment for elevated glucose

The US Preventive Services Task Force recommended *against* routine screening using the EBCT scan (heart scan) because of a lack of evidence that widespread screening could improve health outcomes, particularly in the face of potential complications from diagnostic procedures from false positive exams.[200] While the test can appear attractive on the surface, it is unclear or even unlikely that it will offer real benefit in a screening modality.[201] A task force from the American College of Cardiology and the American Heart Association had similar reservations.[202] They did not support the routine use of the heart scan as a screening tool over and above the traditional use of risk factors.[202] They did offer that if an asymptomatic individual had an intermediate risk (10% to 20% by Framingham calculation), then a positive scan may indicate that the individual should be considered in the high-risk category instead.

In patients with known coronary disease, as well, efforts to use the calcium score from the EBCT scan have not been useful in monitoring the progression of coronary artery disease or its response to statin therapy.[203,204]

Therefore, under current circumstances, the benefit of screening with the EBCT heart scan is unclear. There is no evidence that the technology offers clear value in directing or following our therapy. Also, we need to remember that scanning asymptomatic patients, while occasionally finding a significant unexpected treatable lesion, can also lead to many false positive lesions. Pursuing those false positive lesions can lead to expensive and potentially dangerous procedures.

Chapter 18

HMG-CoA Reductase Inhibitors (Statins)

The HMG-CoA reductase inhibitors, or "statins," as they are commonly called, have revolutionized the preventive treatment of cardiovascular disease. The original discovery was developed from fungi, of a strain similar to the fungi that led to penicillin.[205] The statins work by inhibiting the production of cholesterol at the HMG-CoA reductase step in cholesterol production. This inhibition decreases the cholesterol level in the hepatocyte cells in the liver, inducing the LDL-C receptors on the hepatocyte surface to increase the rate of uptake of LDL from the plasma, thus lowering the

LDL-C concentration in the bloodstream. This action leads to a resetting of the LDL-C regulation by the hepatocyte to a lower serum LDL-C level.[205]

Prior to the development of these agents, there had been controversy about the benefit of medication treatment to lower cholesterol. Once the statins had been studied extensively, the research on their usefulness ended that debate. The data, which will be presented shortly, have overwhelmingly proven that statin treatment not only lowers cholesterol but also reduces all types of cardiac events, including total mortality. In fact, the improvement in cardiac events with statin treatment is so dramatic that many authors wonder if statins have other properties beyond improving the lipid levels that may further reduce heart attack and other cardiac events, commonly referred to as the "pleiotropic" effect. The pleiotropic effect could include anti-inflammatory effects, along with other properties not yet understood.[206]

EVIDENCE OF EFFICACY

The statins have a record of extremely successful research trials that clearly proved their success in preventing a range of cardiovascular events—initial MI, recurrent MI, stroke, cardiovascular death, and even total mortality. This record of success is unmatched by any other medication class. Indeed, beginning with the 4S trial (Scandinavian Simvastatin Survival Study), which showed a very impressive reduction in total mortality from a single medication, all of the statins currently on the market have demonstrated impressive, even incredible effectiveness, in reducing cardiovascular events. Because of the numerous trials supporting the efficacy of the statins, I will only highlight some of the critical trials in this section.

Secondary Prevention

Secondary prevention trials are trials in high-risk patients who have known cardiovascular disease or its equivalent. The original trial is the 4S trial. This trial in Scandinavia treated 4444 men and women with known angina or previous MI along with elevated cholesterol, with either placebo or simvastatin 20 to 40 mg. Total mortality was reduced in the simvastatin patients by 30%, along with a 42% reduction in coronary mortality, a 37% reduction in nonfatal MI, and a 30% reduction in stroke.[207] Two pravastatin trials quickly followed. In the LIPID study, 9014 men and women with known CHD and elevated cholesterol were treated with pravastatin 40 mg or placebo.[208] Pravastatin treatment reduced total mortality 22%, MI 29%, death from coronary disease 25%, and stroke 19%. In the CARE study, 4159 patients with *average*, or *mid-range,* cholesterol and CHD were randomized to pravastatin 40 mg or placebo.[209] While total or coronary mortality were not reduced, pravastatin therapy did reduce MI death and nonfatal MI by 24%, along with reductions in coronary artery bypass grafting (CABG) of 26%, in angioplasty of 23%, and in stroke of 31%.

Fluvastatin 80 mg was studied versus placebo in 1677 patients who had average cholesterol levels but who had just undergone PCI, or percutaneous coronary intervention.[210] Fluvastatin therapy reduced myocardial events by 22% over 4 years. The GRACE study was an observational study that followed 19,537 patients who presented with acute coronary syndrome at hospitals around the world.[211] The study found that patients who arrived on statin therapy with acute coronary syndrome were less likely to have ST-segment elevation or MI, and those acute coronary syndrome patients who continued their statin in the hospital had fewer complications or death.

Of extraordinary importance was the Heart Protection Study out of the United Kingdom.[212] This study enrolled 20,536 British men and women based not on their baseline cholesterol, but on their cardiac risk, with patients having known coronary artery disease, cerebrovascular or peripheral vascular disease, or diabetes. They were randomized to either simvastatin 40 mg or placebo and were followed for 5 years. There were dramatic reductions in many different endpoints in the simvastatin-treated group: total mortality down 12.9%; coronary mortality down 18%; nonfatal or fatal MI down 25%; and a 25% reduction in stroke. Most interestingly, the benefit was seen across all the patient groups, regardless of the baseline cholesterol values, indicating that all high-risk patients should be treated with a statin, regardless of their cholesterol. This remarkable finding has tremendously expanded the number of patients who need statin treatment. Also, there did not appear to be a threshold of "too low" for on-treatment LDL seen in the patients. The HPS study, as it is known, documents that the widespread and aggressive use of statin therapy will reduce cardiac events dramatically, and this study led to new guidelines that recommended this dramatic expansion of treatment.

When all of these secondary prevention trials are considered together, aggressive statin therapy is now mandatory for all patients with atherosclerotic disease of the coronary artery, cerebrovascular arteries, or peripheral arteries, or with diabetes mellitus.

Primary Prevention

Primary prevention trials are those that study individuals who have elevated risk for cardiovascular disease but have not yet developed clinical or symptomatic disease.

The original statin primary prevention trial was the West of Scotland Study.[213] WOSCOPS, as it is also known, randomized 6595 Scottish men with an average LDL-C of 192 mg/dL, but without coronary disease, to either pravastatin 40 mg or placebo. The pravastatin group had a statistically significant 31% reduction in first MI and a 28% reduction in fatal MI, along with a 22% reduction in total mortality (which was of borderline statistical significance). These results were extraordinary, especially when compared to the previous primary prevention trials with other classes of agents. A recently published long-term follow-up from this study showed that the benefit to the pravastatin group persisted for 10 years after the study, with reduced rates of cardiovascular death and total mortality in the group that had received pravastatin for 5 years during the study.[214]

The previously mentioned AFCAPS/TexCAPS was a US primary prevention trial that enrolled patients without previous coronary disease who had mid-range LDL-C (130–190 mg/dL) but with HDL-C < 45 mg/dL for men and < 47 mg/dL for women. The 6605 patients included both men and women and various ethnic minorities. They were randomized to lovastatin 20 to 40 mg or placebo for 5 years.[162] The overall study showed a reduction of 37% in overall cardiac events. A secondary evaluation of this trial demonstrated that most of the events reduction benefit was seen in the patients with HDL-C < 40 mg/dL, where the events reduction was nearly 50%.[163] This secondary analysis shows that statin therapy is an effective treatment in patients with low HDL-C syndrome.

PROSPER was a study in patients aged 70 to 82 years who had either high risks of coronary disease or had previous coronary events.[215] The study enrolled 5804 patients and randomized them to pravastatin 40 mg or placebo, for a total of 5 years. All coronary events were reduced in the pravastatin patients by 15%, including a 24% reduction in cardiac mortality. This study extends the benefit of statin therapy into the very elderly, since patients as old as 87 years were involved in the treatment.

ASCOT-LLA is a cholesterol treatment arm of the ASCOT blood pressure study. The LLA arm randomized 10,305 men and women with elevated cholesterol to atorvastatin 10 mg or placebo.[216] The study was stopped early at 3.3 years because of dramatic reductions of 36% of fatal and nonfatal MIs in the atorvastatin-treated patients, along with a 27% stroke reduction and 21% reduction in total cardiovascular events. The most interesting thing about this study is that the atorvastatin 10 mg dose produced a dramatic 35% reduction in LDL-C but *no change* in the HDL-C, in contrast to other statin trials where HDL-C is increased. This study seems to confirm the strength of the "LDL-C hypothesis," where the reduction in LDL-C produced a clear proportionate reduction in MI.

ALLHAT was the only statin trial that did not demonstrate a clear benefit for reduced cardiac events.[217] However, the design of the study was so flawed that the data is not considered valid.[218] Basically a hypertension trial, ALLHAT had a cholesterol arm where patients were given pravastatin 40 mg, *but versus usual care, not placebo*. So many of the usual-care patients were placed on cholesterol lowering therapy that the LDL-C and other lipid values between the groups were too small to produce a clear benefit. Therefore, this trial is not regarded as significant. In the MEGA study in elderly Japanese women, pravastatin 10 to 20 mg reduced cardiovascular events by 25% for CHD, 37% for stroke, and 41% for total mortality.[219] However, because of the small number of total events in this low-risk population, the reductions did not achieve statistical significance.

The CARDS study was a primary prevention study in patients with type II diabetes mellitus. Patients with diabetes (2838 total), low to normal LDL-C, and no evidence of heart disease, were randomized to atorvastatin 10 mg or placebo.[220] The atorvastatin-treated patients had a 37% reduction in cardiovascular events, a 36% reduction in acute coronary events, and a 48% reduction in stroke. As in ASCOT, the events reduction was all driven by the LDL-C reduction, since the HDL-C was unchanged.

Finally, the previously mentioned JUPITER study showed dramatic reduction in all cardiovascular endpoints when patients with LDL-C < 130 mg/dL but with moderately elevated hs-CRP of > 2mg/dL were given rosuvastatin 20 mg versus placebo.[154] These are the most dramatic reductions seen in any primary prevention trial, and JUPITER could lead to more aggressive lowering of LDL-C, potentially lowering our LDL-C treatment targets to < 70 mg/dL for all patients, or to more frequent use of hs-CRP in screening.

When all the evidence is taken together, there is no doubt about the effectiveness of statin therapy to reduce all forms of cardiovascular events—initial and recurrent MI, cardiovascular death, stroke, and even total mortality—in patients across the range of cholesterol values.

LDL-C Levels

The final statin efficacy question is "How low should our LDL-C target be?" The first evidence came from the Heart Protection Study, which treated patients with simvastatin 40 mg regardless of their baseline LDL-C.[212] Patients whose baseline, and therefore on-treatment LDL-C levels were in the lower third of the baseline values had a lower overall risk of events than did patients with higher baseline and therefore higher on-treatment LDL-C, indicating that there was no lower level for LDL-C where further lowering would not produce further reductions in events. Several studies were undertaken to treat patients to different levels of LDL-C, either by comparing statins of differing potency or by using different doses of the same statin. In general, these studies gave a uniform answer that "the lower the LDL-C, the better off the patients."

PROVE-IT studied patients with acute coronary syndrome, randomizing 4162 men and women to pravastatin 40 mg versus atorvastatin 80 mg.[221] On those treatments, the pravastatin patients achieved the target LDL-C at that time of < 100 mg/dL with an average LDL-C of 95 mg/dL, while the atorvastatin patients achieved an LDL-C of 62 mg/dL. The atorvastatin patients had a 16% reduction in recurrent cardiac events compared to the pravastatin patients. The TNT study randomized 10,001 patients with known coronary disease to atorvastatin 10 mg or atorvastatin 80 mg.[222] The atorvastatin 80 mg patients had an LDL-C of 77 mg/dL, and had a 22% reduction in cardiac events from the atorvastatin 10 mg patients, who had an LDL-C of 101 mg/dL.

Two other comparison studies were not as conclusive as the first 2 but did provide support for more complete LDL-C lowering. In IDEAL, nearly 9000 patients with recent MI were assigned to atorvastatin 80 mg or simvastatin 20 mg.[223] In the simvastatin group, the on-treatment LDL-C was 104 mg/dL while the atorvastatin patients' LDL-C was 81 mg/dL. There was a strong 11% reduction that was of borderline significance ($P = .07$) in major coronary events in the atorvastatin group, with significant reductions in secondary endpoints of 17% in nonfatal MI and 16% in major coronary events. The A to Z trial treated acute coronary patients with either an immediate and high-dose simvastatin regimen of 40 mg/day followed by a titration to 80 mg/day, or a delayed and lower-dose simvastatin regimen of placebo for 4 months and then 20 mg/day.[224] Early events reduction in the higher-dose group compared to the lower dose group was positive at 11% but non-significant. However, from 4 months (when the high-dose titration to simvastatin 80 mg occurred) until the study ended after 3 years, there was a powerful 25% event reduction in the high-dose group.

When all of these studies are evaluated comprehensively, I think there is very clear evidence that using statin therapy to drive the LDL-C down as far as reasonably possible, preferably to the new high-risk target of < 70 mg/dL, and not being satisfied with modest reduction to just < 100 mg/dL, is appropriate and even critical for good patient care. The support for "lower is better" for LDL-C treatment is very clear. Whether we should be aiming for *all* our patients to be treated to a very low LDL-C and whether the target LDL-C should be in the 55 mg/dL range as in JUPITER remains to be seen.

AGENTS AND DOSAGE

There are currently 6 statins available on the US market. All 6 have been shown in at least 1 clinical trial to reduce cardiac events, so there is consensus that the benefits of statins are "class effect," meaning the benefits can be expected from any of the statins. The 6 statins are:

Lovastatin, originally Mevacor, now generic

Pravastatin, originally Pravachol, now generic

Simvastatin, originally Zocor, now generic

Table 18-1 HMG-CoA Reductase Inhibitors—Statins

Agent	Doses	LDL↓	HDL↑	Trig↓
Lovastatin	10, 20, 40, (80) mg	21–32%	5–8%	13–19%[225]
Pravastatin	10, 20, 40, (80) mg	20–30%	3–6%	8–13%[226]
Simvastatin	5, 10, 20, 40, 80 mg	26–45%	5–7%	12–18%[227]
Fluvastatin	20, 40, 80(XL) mg	22–36%	3–7%	12–19%[228]
Atorvastatin	10, 20, 40, 80 mg	39–60%	5–9%	19–37%[229]
Rosuvastatin	5, 10, 20, 40 mg	45–63%	8–13%	23–35%[230]

Fluvastatin, Lescol
Atorvastatin, Lipitor
Rosuvastatin, Crestor

The doses and the expected effects on the lipid fraction are listed in Table 18-1.

There are some differences in regard to dosing within the class. The original 4 statins—lovastatin, pravastatin, simvastatin, and fluvastatin—all have relatively short half-lives, so they need to be taken at *bedtime*, since the body manufactures cholesterol during sleep. Fluvastatin does have an extended release dose in the 80 mg dose only, which can be taken at any time in the day. The 2 newer statins, atorvastatin (Lipitor) and rosuvastatin (Crestor) both have longer half-lives and can be administered once daily at any time in the day.

Also, while the official literature shows that atorvastatin (Lipitor) raises HDL-C somewhat in short-term studies, long-term use of the agent frequently shows either no change in HDL-C or even a reduction.[220]

Choosing the initial dose of a statin is very different from initiating other therapies, like hypertension. One should determine the LDL-C of the patient and the percentage reduction needed to reach the LDL-C target. Then the proper agent and dose should be selected. With the older, less potent statins (lovastatin, pravastatin, simvastatin, and fluvastatin), it is typical to go right to a significant dose, like 40 mg, as initial therapy. There are, however, certain dosing precautions that should be observed. Since statin side effects are frequently dose related, there are certain groups who should have lower initial doses and cautious titration. Elderly patients, small muscle mass patients, and patients with renal compromise should all be dosed cautiously, usually started on lower initial doses and titrated cautiously, always staying below the maximal dose. Since side effects are often driven by the milligram of the dose of statin, in patients where caution is appropriate, a small dose of a more potent statin, say 5 mg of rosuvastatin or 10 mg of atorvastatin will produce more potent LDL-C lowering with less risk of side effects than 40 mg of a less potent statin like simvastatin.

Caution is needed in the treatment of patients of East Asian ancestry (Japanese, Chinese, Korean, Filipino), since individuals from these backgrounds have slower metabolism of statins. This slower metabolism means they should be treated with much lower doses of statin to avoid drug accumulation and toxicity. This protocol has been best defined with rosuvastatin, but it should be applied to all of the statins.

SIDE EFFECTS AND STATIN SAFETY

There has always been concern in the public and the medical community about potential safety problems with the statins. A careful review of the data shows that this concern is unfounded. Overall, the statins are extremely safe, actually safer than many of our over-the-counter preparations. Acetaminophen is a much greater risk for liver failure, as is niacin, both of which are sold over the counter. Non-steroidal anti-inflammatory drugs (NSAIDs) can raise blood pressure and lead to renal damage, which are not seen with the statins. Practitioners and the public need to remember that the mild and limited side effects of statins are more than offset by the tremendous reduction they produce in the leading cause of death and disease—cardiovascular events.

Muscle Side Effects

Statins can clearly cause muscle side effects. These are generally mild and self-limited. There are more serious muscle side effects, but they are quite uncommon. The most serious muscle condition, rhabdomyolysis, while very serious and potentially fatal, is also extremely rare. The definitions and criteria for muscle side effects are listed in Table 18-2.

Table 18-2 Muscle Side Effects of Statins

Condition	Criteria	Evaluation
Myalgia	Muscle aches without significant CK elevation	Consider discontinuation and rechallenge with low-dose of very potent statin.
Myopathy	Muscle pain with CK elevated 10 times normal	Stop statin. Evaluate for other cause of muscle breakdown. Consider muscle biopsy.
Rhabdomyolysis	Marked muscle pain with very high CK; possible renal failure; urine dip + blood, but no RBCs on micro	Refer for admission as an emergency. Consider other causes of muscle breakdown.

Myalgia

Myalgia, or muscle discomfort without objective findings of muscle breakdown, is the most common side effect of statins. The real rate of this is actually quite low, probably in the 2% to 3% range, if it is properly evaluated. Statin myalgia is clinically very similar to polymyalgia rheumatica. It is a bilateral condition, usually affecting the large muscle groups like both shoulder girdles, both thighs, or the upper back. The bilateral nature of it is the key to making the proper diagnosis. If the discomfort is unilateral, it is attributable to some other process, not the statin. Also, it is not *joint* pain, which is arthralgia. It is *muscle* pain, which is different than joint pain. Since most patients do not discriminate between joint and muscle pain, a careful history and exam of the muscle that might be involved is crucial.

Be very cautious about overdiagnosing statins as the cause of the routine aches and pains of adult life. Statins are lifesaving therapy and many of the aches and pains that patients have are not caused by their statins but are just the routine aches and pains of advancing age. In the recent JUPITER study, 16% of the rosuvastatin and 15.4% of the placebo patients had muscle symptoms, which is essentially no difference.[158] Similar reports are found in many other studies. Therefore, approach this diagnosis carefully. We do not want to stop potentially lifesaving medication because of routine aches and pains.

Myopathy

Myopathy is a much more serious condition. Myopathy is defined as muscle pain with a creatine kinase (CK) elevated to 10 times above the normal level. The muscles are usually somewhat tender. Statin myopathy is rare, with 10 cases seen in the 10,000 patients who received simvastatin 40 mg in the Heart Protection Study. In the Heart Protection Study, 4 of the 10,000 patients on placebo also had myopathy, probably idiopathic in nature, with a placebo myopathy rate of about half that seen in the patients on simvastatin.[212] In the A to Z trial, the rate of myopathy on simvastatin 80 mg was 5 times greater than the rate on 40 mg in the Heart Protection Study, at 5 cases per 1000 patients, which must have been produced by the higher 80 mg dose of simvastatin.[224]

If a patient has muscle symptoms and a CK elevation in the area of > 10 times normal (or even lower), stop the statin at once and monitor their renal function. If their renal status is unaffected, then you have time for an outpatient evaluation. You should evaluate them for other inflammatory conditions that can cause myopathy, like polymyositis. Since statins are frequently critically important therapy, a muscle biopsy may be indicated to determine if the myopathy is related to the statin or not, since statin myopathy does have a particular cellular pattern seen on the biopsy.

Rhabdomyolysis

Rhabdomyolysis is the most serious muscle condition seen with the statins. Rhabdomyolysis can be a life-threatening condition that requires emergency referral for admission. Rhabdomyolysis presents as marked muscle pain, often with systemic symptoms. Muscle pain and breakdown are severe. The CK levels are usually markedly elevated. The muscle breakdown can be so severe that excess myoglobin in the bloodstream can lead to renal shutdown. The myoglobin can produce dark urine that is dipstick positive for blood (from the globin molecule) but has no red blood cells present on microscopic exam. Renal shutdown from the excessive muscle breakdown may actually require dialysis.

Rhabdomyolysis is very rare, and the FDA database reports that the risk of fatal rhabdomyolysis caused by statin monotherapy is about 1 case in 7 million statin prescriptions annually.[231] This risk is about equal to the risk of flying on a commercial airliner. When this risk is compared to the risk of dying from untreated cholesterol elevation, it is clear that the statins are very safe and beneficial. Many cases of rhabdomyolysis involve drug interactions, underlying medical problems, or inappropriate dosing. Table 18-3 lists many of the underlying conditions that increase the risk of muscle problems. Muscle problems in statin therapy are frequently multifactorial. If fact, many of the more serious muscle problems associated with statin therapy are interactions with other problems. These are highlighted in Table 18-3.

Finally, we should all be very cautious about the 80 mg dose of statin. In general, I avoid the 80 mg dose, going to a more potent statin instead.[158] The best evaluations of statin muscle and liver problems are Bryan Brewer's evaluations, which are presented in Figure 18-1 and Figure 18-2. They clearly show that the main drivers for increased rates of significant myopathy and liver enzyme elevations are the 80 mg doses currently in use.[232] Therefore, I have recommended that one of the easier ways to reduce the risk of statin side effects is to get comfortable with using the more potent statins, rosuvastatin and atorvastatin.[158,233] With their more potent lowering of LDL-C, you can frequently achieve the LDL-C target with a lower dose, thus reducing the risk of muscle problems or other side effects.

Table 18-3 Factors That Increase the Risk of Statin-Related Myopathy

Drug Interactions

- Gemfibrozil should not be used with any statin
- Fenofibrate should be used with caution
- Cytochrome P-450 3A4 agents—avoid with lovastatin, simvastatin, and atorvastatin
- Azole antifungals
- Cyclosporine
- Grapefruit juice
- HIV Protease inhibitors
- Macrolide antibiotics (i.e., erythromycin, clarithromycin)
- Nefazodone
- Verapamil
- Diltiazem
- Niacin
- Warfarin

Patient Conditions

- Advanced age (particularly thin, frail, older women)
- Alcohol abuse
- Major surgery
- Multiple medications
- Multisystem disease (e.g., chronic renal insufficiency, especially due to diabetes)

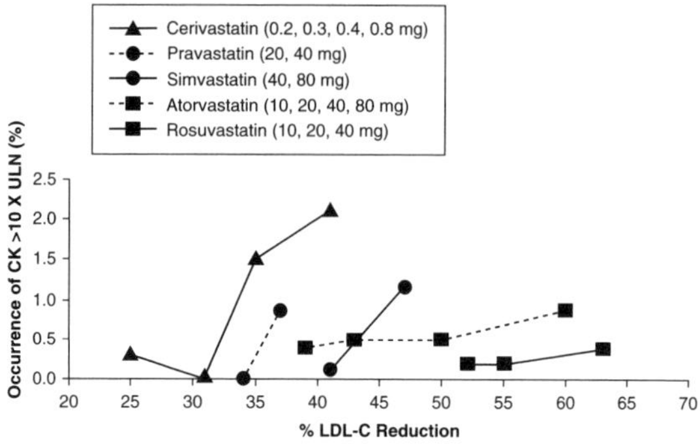

Figure 18-1 Relationship of Statin Dose, LDL-C Reduction, and Myopathy
Source: **Copyright © 2003 Excerpta Medica Inc. All rights reserved.**

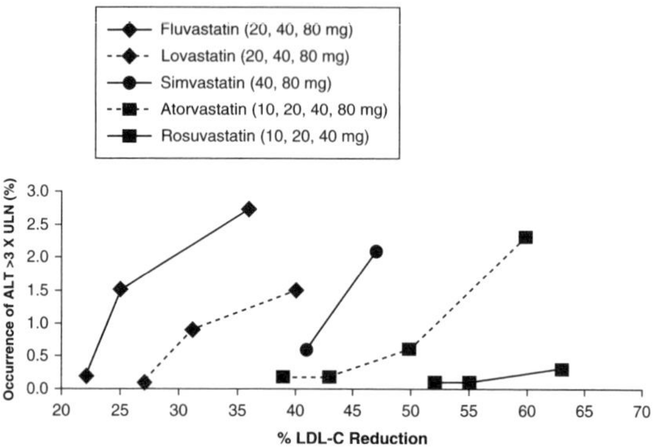

Figure 18-2 Relationship of Statin Dose, LDL-C Reduction, and Liver Enzyme Elevations
Source: **Copyright © 2003 Excerpta Medica Inc. All rights reserved.**

Liver Safety

It was noticed from the early days of the development of the statins that some patients would have elevated levels of liver enzymes in the blood. There was, therefore, a concern that the statins may have some risk of liver toxicity. This had led to recommendations for a regular monitoring for elevated liver enzymes and possible cessation if persistently high levels of liver enzymes are detected.

There appears to be much confusion as to how much risk of liver toxicity there is with statin therapy and what constitutes a significant elevation. Broadly accepted guidelines are as follows:

- Monitor liver enzymes at baseline, before starting therapy.
- Recheck at 12 weeks, then every 6 months thereafter.
- Monitor for ALT/AST (alanine aminotransferase and aspartate aminotransferase) > 3 times normal on 2 successive measurements before considering cessation of statin.

Recently, many academicians have come to feel that the concern about potential liver risk from statins has been overstated.[234] Examining the pivotal clinical trials with statins—4S, WOSCOPS, AFCAPS/TexCAPS, HPS, and JUPITER—shows no significant difference in the rate of liver enzyme elevations at the > 3 times normal on consecutive specimens between the statin and the placebo groups.[154,162,207,212,213,234] Further analyses of the statin trials also found insignificant rates of liver enzyme elevations.[235,236]

Other lipid-lowering medications have also been shown to have similar rates of liver enzyme elevations. Ezetimibe has a completely different mechanism for reducing lipid fractions, as do the bile acid resins, but each has similar rates of liver enzyme elevations as seen in the statin trials.[236,237] These mild, inconsistent liver enzyme elevations may very well not indicate actual damage to the hepatocyte cells of the liver, but simply an alteration in the permeability of cellular membranes, allowing a leak of the enzymes without damage to the hepatocyte, a condition called "transaminitis" by one author, in contrast to statin hepatitis.[238]

The fundamental question is whether statin therapy is associated with major liver damage, rather than just minor enzyme leaks. A careful study of the cases of liver transplantation for acute drug-induced liver failure in the United States between 1990 and 2002 concluded that statins did not cause liver failure. During that 12-year period, 1 case of liver failure was attributed to simvastatin, a rate so low that it probably was an "idiopathic" case of liver failure in a person who happened to be taking a statin.[239] Two other cases were attributed to cerivastatin, but that agent has been removed from the market. Other authors have studied this question and concluded that the rate of liver failure in patients taking statins is lower than the "baseline" rate of idiopathic liver failure in the general population.[240–242] This conclusion is recognized by a statement from an ACC/AHA/NHLBI panel on statin safety.[243] The lack of evidence of clear statin liver injury has led several authors and the National Lipid Association to conclude that routine monitoring of liver enzymes does not increase patient safety and may actually lead to unnecessary discontinuation of appropriate therapy in some individuals. [244–246]

Despite all these questions about the value of monitoring liver enzymes, the recommendation for regular monitoring remains in place. Therefore, for medical/legal reasons, practitioners should continue regular routine monitoring. However, minor elevations in liver enzymes should be treated with caution. Again, significant elevations are > 3 times the normal AST/ALT levels, and they must be seen on 2 consecutive tests. If they are detected at that level, an investigation should consider other etiologies, such as viral infection (hepatitis A, B, or C); alcohol abuse; other medications, including over-the-counter preparations like acetaminophen and NSAIDs, and alternative therapies.[241,244] While discontinuation of statin therapy may be necessary, a careful examination of these questions should be undertaken first.

Renal Safety

There had not been a pattern of concern about potential renal toxicity from statin therapy until the marketing of rosuvastatin (Crestor), when a slightly higher rate of proteinuria on the rosuvastatin 40 mg dose was noted. A careful evaluation of the data in the rosuvastatin question concluded that there was no evidence of renal toxicity for rosuvastatin or any of the statins, outside of the very rare rhabdomyolysis cases.[247] A comprehensive report from the FDA in 2005 found that there was no evidence of renal toxicity from rosuvastatin and that the dipstick proteinuria was not an indicator of glomerular damage or renal decline.[248]

The mild and inconsistent leaks of urinary protein come from tubular origins, not from the glomerulus, and they are produced by inhibition of the HMG-CoA reductase system for reabsorption of tubular protein secretion.[249,250] Therefore, this mild proteinuria is inconsequential and not indicative of renal damage.

Indeed, several authors have documented that statins appear to protect renal function, in a fashion similar to the ACE inhibitors. Statins have been shown to reduce glomerular proteinuria and to protect or even slightly improve renal function across the statin class, including rosuvastatin.[249–257] Therefore, statins should not be considered potentially renal toxic.

STATIN THERAPY QUESTIONS

Are statins effective in women?

Yes. While the original statin trials were dominated by male patients, there have been considerable numbers of female patients in the subsequent studies. Overall, women had the same benefit pattern as men across the various studies. The most recent study, JUPITER, is a good example. In JUPITER, 38% of the patients were female, and the response rate for women was equivalent to men.[154] Therefore, women should not be denied appropriate statin therapy, since the potential benefit is expected to be the same for them as for men.

Statins, however, have never been studied in pregnancy situations, so everyone acknowledges that they should not be used in fertile females. In the rare situations where a fertile female requires lipid-lowering therapy, most physicians should refer this rare but difficult problem to a lipid specialist.

Can we drive the LDL-C too low with statins?

This is an excellent question, particularly as we see studies like JUPITER driving LDL-C lower and lower. There clearly should be a "too low" LDL-C threshold, but nobody has identified it yet. Therefore, any attempt to identify it is educated guesswork.

What evidence we do have comes from the long-term treatment trials. Many of these trials, like JUPITER, 4S, PROVE-IT, and TNT, have had some of their patients down into the LDL-C levels of the low 40 mg/dL's and even the high 30 mg/dL's. None of these studies have been able to identify a "too low" threshold.

In general, I am delighted to treat my patients' LDLs down into the 50 mg/dL's, and I am comfortable with them in the mid 40 mg/dL's range. If they drop into the 30 mg/dL's, then

I back down on the therapy. I am comfortable with this approach, but I cannot say it has been proven safe. However, I do know that reducing LDL-C in vulnerable patients has been shown to reduce their risk of CHD dramatically. We need to remember that we do not want to undertreat patients and allow their LDL to be higher than it should be out of a concern that an LDL-C in, say the high 40 mg/dL's *might* be a problem later.

Do I need to start statins at their lowest dose and then titrate up, like we frequently do in hypertension?

No. Many of the statin trials have started the patients on the maximum dose that was recommended at the time, like pravastatin 40 mg (WOSCOPS, CARE, LIPID), simvastatin 40 mg (HPS), or rosuvastatin 20 mg (JUPITER). I would recommend that you evaluate each patient and choose the appropriate agent and dose that is appropriate for his or her baseline and target LDL-C. Remember that there are specific groups—East Asians, patients with small body size, patients with renal compromise, and the very elderly—for whom smaller initial and even therapeutic doses are necessary.

With patients requiring a dramatic LDL-C reduction, I think it is best to go right to an appropriate dose of one of the more potent statins, like rosuvastatin or atorvastatin, to avoid a lengthy titration process.

What is the "rule of six"?

The "rule of six" is that you can expect to see a further reduction of LDL-C by only an additional 6% each time you double the statin dose. For example, if you see a 20% LDL-C reduction with a dose of pravastatin of 20 mg, increasing it to 40 mg will only reduce the LDL-C to a total of 26%. This rule applies to all of the statins and all of the doses.

Therefore, going from the 40 mg dose to the 80 mg dose of any of the statins, while greatly increasing the risk of muscle or liver side effects, will only generate a further 6% reduction of LDL-C. This is why I recommend that all practitioners get comfortable with using atorvastatin and rosuvastatin, our most potent statins, as our LDL-C targets continue to drop lower and lower.

What are the most likely drug interactions with statins?

The most severe and likely drug interaction is between gemfibrozil and all of the statins. Gemfibrozil inhibits the glucuronidation pathway of statin metabolism, often leading to toxic levels of statin and rhabdomyolysis.[231] Indeed, gemfibrozil/statin interaction has been a significant contributor to rhabdomyolysis cases reported to the FDA, including many of the fatal cases.[231] There appears to be much less of a risk with the use of fenofibrate instead of gemfibrozil.[231] However, practitioners need to be aware that it has never been shown that adding a fibrate to statin therapy further reduces cardiovascular risk. People assume that the combination will be beneficial, but that has not been proven. Therefore, I *never* use gemfibrozil at all, and I currently do not add fenofibrate to a statin. Others do, but I do not.

Three of the statins, lovastatin, simvastatin, and atorvastatin, are metabolized through the CYP450 3A4 system, making them vulnerable to toxicity if they are used with agents that inhibit that system. Those agents are listed in Table 18-3.

Has it been proven that adding a second lipid-lowering agent to a statin reduces cardiac events more than the statin alone?

No. There are several products combining a statin with a second cholesterol agent on the market now, with others to follow. Also, some prescribers frequently add second agents to a statin to raise HDL-C or to lower triglycerides. None of these combinations have been shown to reduce cardiac events more than the statin alone.

This matter will be covered further in other areas in the text, but at this point there is no evidence, just assumptions, that combining a second agent with a statin will result in further events reduction than the statin alone.

SUMMARY

In summary, the statins have been comprehensively studied and proven to reduce all aspects of cardiovascular events—initial MI, recurrent MI, stroke, cardiovascular mortality, and total mortality—across the spectrum of patients. The statins are extremely safe, with very rare significant side effects. Therefore, the statins are always the initial choice for treatment of LDL-C elevation and low HDL-C cholesterol disorders. The other agents must be considered in a secondary role behind the statins.

Chapter 19
Ezetimibe

Ezetimibe is a widely used agent for the reduction of LDL-C. It is currently the only agent in its class and works by inhibiting absorption of cholesterol in the small intestine. The area of action is at the sterol transporter in the small intestine at a site designated the NPC1L1.[258,259]

Ezetimibe in its 10 mg dose lowers LDL-C by 18 mg/dL, raises HDL-C by 1 mg/dL, and lowers triglycerides by 8 mg/dL. Ezetimibe is marketed alone as Zetia, but its relatively modest LDL-C lowering has meant that most of its use has been in combination with simvastatin as Vytorin. Vytorin is currently marketed in 4 combinations:

Vytorin 10/10—ezetimibe 10 mg and simvastatin 10 mg
Vytorin 10/20—ezetimibe 10 mg and simvastatin 20 mg
Vytorin 10/40—ezetimibe 10 mg and simvastatin 40 mg
Vytorin 10/80—ezetimibe 10 mg and simvastatin 80 mg

The improvements in lipid fractions are shown in Table 19-1.

Table 19-1 Lipid Effects from Vytorin Doses

Vytorin Dose	Total-C	LDL-C	HDL-C	Trig
Vytorin 10/10	−31%	−45%	+8%	−23%
Vytorin 10/20	−36%	−52%	+10%	−24%
Vytorin 10/40	−39%	−55%	+6%	−23%
Vytorin 10/80	−43%	−60%	+6%	−31%

Ezetimibe has been studied as additive therapy with statins other than simvastatin. It shows the same degree of additive changes with the other statins as it does with simvastatin.

EVIDENCE OF EFFICACY

The fundamental question about ezetimibe has been, and remains, the complete lack of evidence that the LDL-C reduction produced by ezetimibe will translate into the expected reduction in cardiovascular events. Ezetimibe has enjoyed considerable sales and financial success since it was introduced based strictly on the *assumption* that the LDL-C reduction produced by ezetimibe will produce the same events reduction as that seen with the statins.[260]

The problem with this approach is that *assumptions are assumptions, not proof*. The issue was not dealt with at the outset of marketing, since ezetimibe was allowed onto the market without proof of its events reduction ability.

Recent data has begun to fuel a controversy about ezetimibe. The ENHANCE trial was the first comprehensive trial comparing the combination of simvastatin 80 mg combined with ezetimibe 10 mg (Vytorin 10/80) against simvastatin 80 mg monotherapy. Over a 2-year period, the trial evaluated 720 patients with familial hypercholesterolemia and baseline LDL-C of 317 to 319 mg/dL. The trial used B-mode ultrasound to evaluate changes in the intimae-media thickness in the carotid and femoral arteries, as a surrogate marker for the progression of atherosclerotic changes. On treatment, the Vytorin group did have a considerably lower LDL-C than the simvastatin group (141 mg/dL vs. 192 mg/dL), but this did not produce improvement in the carotid intima, actually showing a non-significant worsening.[261]

This trial has generated considerable discussion about the value of ezetimibe therapy. Authors have urged caution about the routine use of ezetimibe, emphasizing that statin therapy should be maximized before adding ezetimibe.[262,263]

The SEAS trial studied 1873 patients with aortic stenosis but without known coronary or other atherosclerotic disease to simvastatin 40 mg plus ezetimibe 10 mg, or placebo, for 4 years. Baseline LDL-C was 139 mg/dL, well above the LDL-C level treated in the JUPITER study. Strangely, this treatment did *not* produce a significant reduction in the primary combined endpoint.[264] There were some trends and reductions in secondary endpoints, but the overall study was unsuccessful. Based on other studies like the Heart Protection Study, I would have expected the simvastatin alone to have produced more improvement in events reduction than the combination did.

Together, I think these 2 studies raise serious questions about the ability of ezetimibe to produce the sort of reduction in cardiac events that its LDL-C reduction would lead us to expect.

Further controversy came from the SEAS trial, where the ezetimibe group was found to have significant increases in cancer deaths and cancer cases.[264] There was, however, no particular pattern to the cancer cases or sites of cancer. A follow-up study compared the SEAS data to 2 other ongoing ezetimibe trials, where there were no increases in cancer cases or deaths.[265] I personally think this issue is simply the result of a chance cluster of cancer patients, since the cases were not of a particular type of tumor or site of tumor, but we do not have clear proof.

A large, ongoing trial called IMPROVE-IT is comparing combined ezetimibe/simvastatin to simvastatin alone to see if the combination reduces cardiac events compared to simvastatin alone. Recently, it was announced that the trial would be expanded from 12,500 patients to 18,000 patients and extended to run through 2012.[266] This alteration in this most pivotal trial has raised the question that ongoing events may not be favorable for the ezetimibe combination, possibly leading the investigators to expand and lengthen the study in an effort to increase its chances of success.

SIDE EFFECTS

The side effects from ezetimibe are quite limited and very mild. There is, as with all lipid-lowering therapies, a low level of elevated liver enzymes and the potential for myopathy changes and even rhabdomyolysis.[258] There are potential drug interactions with warfarin and cyclosporine, and cautions in renal failure patients.

SUMMARY

Ezetimibe is a widely used agent that has not yet been shown to reduce cardiovascular events. My personal recommendation is that it should not be used routinely and certainly not until the patient has been on the maximal tolerated statin therapy. In my practice, I use it in addition to rosuvastatin 40 mg or a lower dose if the 40 mg dose is not tolerated. I advise the patients that the addition will lower their LDL-C considerably but that I do not know if it will lower their heart attack risk.

Chapter 20

The Fibrates (Fibric Acid Derivatives)

There are currently 2 fibrates, or fibric acid derivatives, on the US market, fenofibrate (TriCor and generic) and gemfibrozil. A third, benzafibrate is on the market in Europe and other countries. Fibrates activate the PPAR (peroxisome proliferator-activated receptor) system, which increases clearance of triglycerides from the serum. This triglyceride reduction alters LDL-C from small dense particles to larger, less dense particles, facilitating their clearance from the serum.

The fibrates have their most significant effect on lipid fractions by lowering triglycerides and raising HDL-C, with more modest effects on LDL-C.

EVIDENCE OF EFFICACY

The fibrates are a complicated group of agents to evaluate. Their events reduction trials show a very mixed record, and many of the trials are decades old and difficult, if not impossible, to place in our modern era along with regular use of statin therapy.

The original fibrate was clofibrate, which was involved in several studies in the 1970s. The Coronary Drug Project was the original cholesterol treatment study. One of its arms evaluated clofibrate in high-risk patients with known CHD. The study did not show a significant reduction in overall or cardiovascular mortality, but only a reduction in nonfatal MI. Because of excess deaths in the non-cardiac group, primarily gastrointestinal or gallbladder in nature, clofibrate has been removed from the US and European markets.

Gemfibrozil has been involved in 2 very important trials, the Helsinki Heart Study and the VA HIT study. The Helsinki Heart Study was a primary prevention trial in Finland that studied 4061 men between ages 40 and 55 years. They were randomized to gemfibrozil 600 mg twice daily or placebo for 5 years. There were modest changes in the lipids, with a 10% reduction in LDL-C, a 10% increase in HDL-C, and a 40% reduction in triglycerides.[133] There was a reduction in cardiac endpoints, driven primarily by a 37% reduction in nonfatal MI. There were no significant reductions in cardiac or total mortality. A further evaluation showed that the events reduction was driven by the increase in the HDL-C, not the reduction in triglycerides.[159] A long-term follow-up after 18 years showed that the gemfibrozil continued to be beneficial during an 18-year extension.[267] Furthermore, this evaluation confirmed that the benefit was seen primarily in patients with metabolic syndrome, with increased body mass index, low HDL-C, and increased triglycerides.

The VA HIT study was a US secondary prevention trial, studying 2531 US male veterans with known heart disease, but LDL-C of 111 mg/dL, HDL-C of 32 mg/dL, and triglycerides of 161 mg/dL.[160] They were randomized to gemfibrozil 600 mg twice daily or placebo, for 5 years. The gemfibrozil had no effect on the LDL-C, while raising HDL-C by 6% and lowering triglycerides by 31%. There was a 22% reduction in nonfatal or fatal MI, with a trend for a reduction in coronary death but no reduction in total mortality. A follow-up study determined that the benefit was produced by the elevation in HDL-C, not the triglyceride reduction.[161] However, both of these studies were completed in the era prior to the appearance of the statins, so their relevance now is unclear.

Fenofibrate is now generic, and there is significant interest in using it in combination with statins. There is limited research on fenofibrate in reducing cardiac events. The largest is the FIELD study. FIELD enrolled a high-risk population, 9795 patients with type II diabetes mellitus, 22% with previous CHD, who were not on statin therapy.[268] Patients were randomized to fenofibrate 200 mg daily or placebo and followed for 5 years. The study, in spite of the high-risk patients, was not successful, with a non-significant 11% reduction in coronary events, including a 24% reduction in nonfatal MI but a non-significant 19% increase in coronary death and a non-significant 17% increase in total mortality.

Finally, benzafibrate was studied in Israel in 3090 patients with known coronary disease and with HDL-C ≤ 45 mg/dL, triglycerides ≤ 300 mg/dL, and LDL-C ≤ 180 mg/dL. After 6.2 years, there was a non-significant reduction in cardiac events or cardiac deaths.[269]

In examining these data, it is clear that evidence for the use of fibrates as monotherapy to prevent CHD is absent at this time. There is, as yet, no clear evidence whether adding a fibrate, specifically fenofibrate, to statin therapy, might improve the events reduction from the statin alone. A fenofibrate/statin combination trial in diabetic patients, ACCORD, is currently underway and will offer some assistance with that question.[270]

There are several combination products currently under development, combining fenofibric acid with statins, with the expectation being that the addition of fenofibric acid might improve a number of the non–LDL-C lipid fractions (HDL-C, triglycerides, non–HDL-C, and others) and that this might improve events reduction. Some preliminary data indicate that the issue may not be completely clear. When fenofibric acid was added to rosuvastatin 10 mg, there were significant improvements in these ratios: total-C/HDL-C, non–HDL-C/HDL-C, ApoB/ApoA1, and triglyceride/HDL-C.[271] However, when fenofibric acid was added to rosuvastatin *20 mg*, the significant improvements were eliminated by the higher dose of rosuvastatin, except for the triglyceride/HDL-C ratio. The fact that the higher statin dose overwhelms the improvement from the fenofibric acid may be quite significant in the future. We will not begin to have clear evidence for the concept of combination therapy until the ACCORD trial is completed.

Because of the significant drug interaction between gemfibrozil and statins, I recommend that gemfibrozil never be administered with a statin.

AGENTS AND DOSAGE

The clear use for the fibrates is Fredrickson types IV and V hypertriglyceride syndromes, where triglycerides are > 300 to 500 mg/dL and often > 1000 mg/dL, and LDL-C is normal. The elevated triglycerides are frequently associated with pancreatitis, even though it is not clear if lowering the triglycerides will prevent pancreatitis. Other treatments for elevated triglycerides include weight loss, exercise, and a low-fat and particularly low-carbohydrate diet.

The impacts of the 2 available fibrates are listed in Table 20-1.

Whether these agents have a place in the treatment of LDL-C elevation syndromes, including Fredrickson type II-A (↑LDL-C with normal HDL-C and normal triglycerides) or type II-B (↑LDL-C, ↓HDL-C, and ↑triglycerides) is unclear at this point and will require further research. I personally do not use gemfibrozil at all out of concern that another practitioner might also put the patient on a statin, resulting in a toxic drug interaction with the gemfibrozil. Therefore, if you are going to use a fibrate, I would recommend fenofibrate. (See Table 20-2.)

Table 20-1 The Impact of the 2 Available Fibrates (Fibric Acid Agents)

Agent	↓Total-C	↓LDL-C	↑HDL-C	↓Trig
Fenofibrate				
Trig 300–500 mg/dL	9%	14.5%	19.6%	46%
Trig > 500 mg/dL	13.8%	45%	22.9%	44%
Gemfibrozil	4–11%	0–10%	6–12%	31–43% (272,133,160)

Table 20-2 Comparison of Fenofibrate and Gemfibrozil

Agent	Doses	Schedule	Cautions
Fenofibrate	48–145 mg	Once daily	Use lower dose in elderly and renal failure. Initiate therapy at 48 mg for all patients.
Gemfibrozil	600 mg	Twice daily	Never use with a statin.

SIDE EFFECTS

The fibrates have a noticeable side effect profile, often with potential problems that overlap with those of the statins. The fibrates are associated with elevated liver enzymes and also with increased gallstones, which are secondary to the increase in triglyceride secretion into the bile.

They are also associated with myopathy and even with rhabdomyolysis, either as monotherapy or especially when added to a statin. While fenofibrate has *less* drug interaction with statins that might lead to toxic levels of statins, it does increase statin levels when they are used together. Therefore, caution and dose adjustment should be used if you feel the need to use fenofibrate and a statin together.[272]

USE OF THE FIBRATES

Fibrates are clearly the agent of choice when dealing with markedly high-triglyceride situations, like Frederickson type IV disorder. Their use as monotherapy for high LDL-C lipid disorders has been eliminated by the tremendous success of the statins in treating LDL-C and even low HDL-C disorders. Their use in combined therapy with statins has potential problems, severe with gemfibrozil, and has not yet been shown to be of benefit in reducing cardiovascular events. Therefore, I urge caution to practitioners. We have no clear evidence that combination fibrate/statin therapy offers benefit above statin therapy alone. I personally plan to wait for clear therapeutic evidence before I consider such combination therapy.

Chapter 21

Niacin

Niacin, or nicotinic acid, is a B-vitamin that has been used as a cholesterol lowering agent for decades. The actual mechanism by which niacin lowers cholesterol is not clearly understood.

Niacin has been available in a wide variety of preparations, with many of them sold over the counter, particularly in the form of shorter acting preparations. Many practitioners prefer to utilize longer acting preparations that are prescription products, such as Niaspan and Slo-Niacin.

My opinion is that, even though niacin is a vitamin and is available over the counter, its use in cholesterol management is complicated by considerable safety issues with niacin that lead me to recommend that it should be utilized by prescription only and monitored carefully by a professional.

EVIDENCE OF EFFICACY

The data about events reduction with niacin therapy have been documented, but those results are not clearly understood. The only clear events trial that evaluated niacin as monotherapy was the Coronary Drug Project published in the 1970s. In the niacin arm of this study, niacin treatment did not reduce total or cardiovascular deaths, but it did have a 36% reduction in nonfatal MI, a secondary endpoint.[130] However, this study used niacin in the doses of 3.0 to 3.5 grams, doses much higher than we use in our current treatment schemes, so the relevance of this information for our current practice patterns is very limited. A follow-up evaluation, conducted 9 years after the study had been completed, found that the group that had received niacin in the study had an 11% reduction in total mortality.[273] However, we need to be cautious not to over-interpret these studies. The reduction in the original study was a limited reduction to a *secondary endpoint only*, not the primary endpoint, which showed *no effect from that very high-dose niacin therapy*. With trial results like that, we cannot draw clear conclusions about benefit when only a secondary endpoint showed positive results. In the follow-up report, the study had been over for 9 years, and the patients had not been treated for those years, so it is not possible to interpret the meaning, if any, of that second report.

Niacin has been involved in a series of combination trials when it was used in conjunction with other cholesterol lowering therapy. The only published events trial with a statin had a niacin/simvastatin compared to antioxidant vitamins, placebo, or a combination of antioxidant vitamins and simvastatin/niacin. Since the study did not have individual simvastatin or niacin monotherapy arms, we cannot tell if the combination would have had increased efficacy versus simvastatin or niacin if they had been taken as monotherapy.[274]

The CLAS study looked at a combined treatment with niacin and colestipol, a resin binder. The study followed patients with previous coronary bypass surgery and evaluated the progression of the previously documented angiographic lesions. The combination therapy did slow progression of arterial lesions but did not produce a significant reduction in events.[275,276] However, the significance of atherosclerotic progression studies like this is not clear, since they did not show any reduction in cardiac events. The only niacin combination study to show cardiac events reduction was a Swedish study also where niacin was added to clofibrate.[277] Since clofibrate is off the market, this study offers us no practical importance.

The AIM-HIGH study, currently combining niacin plus simvastatin versus simvastatin alone for cardiovascular events, is being conducted by the National Heart, Lung, and Blood Institute of the National Institutes of Health.[278] When completed, the study should offer insight into whether, and when, niacin/statin combination therapy might be useful.

AGENTS AND DOSAGE

Niacin comes in so many preparations and doses, both over the counter and by prescription, that a complete listing of them is not reasonable. Because most practitioners use one of the prescription preparations, I will focus on them.

Slo-Niacin is a generic preparation designed for a once- (or potentially twice-) a-day use, and it has dose preparations of 250 mg, 500 mg, and 750 mg.

Niaspan is a once-a-day prescription preparation, designed for a bedtime dosage, and it has 500 mg, 750 mg, and 1000 mg preparations.

Dosing niacin preparations requires monitoring and individualization of therapy. In general, one should start at the initial doses, like the 500 mg dose of Niaspan taken at bedtime, then titrate by gradually increasing doses after at least 4 weeks, trying to lessen the side effects, which are often considerable.

The effects of niacin on the various lipid fractions vary considerably with the dose. In general, lipid responses to low doses of 1000 mg or less are mainly a 10% to 15% increase in HDL-C, with minimal reduction in LDL-C and triglyceride levels. When doses are considerably higher, in the 2000 mg range, the HDL-C increase is about 20%, with LDL-C reductions of about 15% and triglyceride reductions of about 30% to 40%.

Therefore, most current clinical use of niacin by practitioners is at lower doses in an effort to increase low HDL-C syndrome, an unproven but popular treatment. Higher doses, in the 1500 to 3000 mg range, are occasionally used as additional therapy in severe LDL-C elevation, as an addition to statin and ezetimibe therapy.

SIDE EFFECTS

The side effects of niacin can be considerable and potentially quite dangerous, particularly for a product that is often taken over the counter.

Liver Dysfunction

Liver dysfunction, often severe and even with fulminant hepatic failure, is the most serious side effect of niacin. It is seen less with the slow-release, prescription preparations if they are begun at low initial doses, even if the patient has been on a much higher dose of immediate release, over-the-counter niacin. Careful monitoring of hepatic enzymes is very important in the administration of niacin. Caution about administering niacin to patients with histories of alcohol abuse or with preexisting liver problems usually will exclude niacin use in those patients. The combination of niacin with other agents with potential liver toxicity, such as fibrates or statins, may require careful monitoring and careful dose adjustment.[279]

Muscle Toxicity

Muscle toxicity, even rhabdomyolysis, can occur with niacin monotherapy. This risk, therefore, is considerably amplified when niacin is added to statins and/or fibrates—agents that have their own risk of muscle toxicity. If any of the cholesterol lowering medications are to be used in combination, patients and practitioners need to be cautious about this combined myopathy risk.

Glucose Metabolism

Glucose metabolism can be negatively affected by niacin therapy. Niacin can worsen control of diabetes and induce glucose intolerance in a number of patients.[280] Since metabolic syndrome, with low HDL-C and elevated triglycerides is commonly present in patients who are candidates for niacin therapy, this side effect risk needs to be considered when initiating or titrating niacin.

Symptomatic Side Effects

Symptomatic, but not dangerous, side effects are common with niacin. Flushing is the most common side effect, and most patients will have some degree of flushing. Some patients do adapt so that the niacin can be continued. Increased flushing is often seen as doses are increased, but there is some evidence that flushing with the time-release preparations may be less than with the immediate release preparations.[281] Many patients find that a dose of aspirin or another NSAID at the time of the niacin dose reduces the flushing, but that is unclear. In my experience, the flushing side effect is more significant than the literature reports, making the use of niacin difficult for many people.

CURRENT USE OF NIACIN

The proper use of niacin in our current treatment pattern is difficult to define, at least until the AIM-HIGH study is reported. Niacin has the potential to significantly increase HDL-C, but the significance of this benefit on top of statin therapy is unclear. Niacin's potential is restricted by its side effect pattern, which can be both uncomfortable (flushing) and/or dangerous (liver or muscle problems). Therefore, cautious and thoughtful use—if any use—should be our guide.

Chapter 22

Bile Acid Sequestrates

The bile acid sequestrates are among the older cholesterol lowering agents. They have been relegated to a very secondary role by the much better efficacy and tolerability of the statins. The bile acid resins are not absorbed in the intestine. They lower cholesterol by forming an insoluble compound with the bile salts that are regularly secreted by the liver into the intestine. This insoluble compound contains cholesterol in the bile salts, and it remains in the intestine and is excreted in the feces.

The use of the bile acid resins, as they are frequently called, has been severely limited in recent years. Since they are confined to the intestines, they can cause considerable abdominal side effects, including abdominal pain, bloating, constipation, and other symptoms. These symptoms are dose related, frequently making it difficult to administer enough dosage to produce effective LDL-C reductions.

EVIDENCE OF EFFICACY

There has been only 1 trial directly evaluating the use of a resin-binding agent for the reduction of cardiac events—LRC-CPPT, a primary prevention trial published in 1984.[132] LRC-CPPT was a 7-year, placebo-controlled study. Cholestyramine was administered at 24 g/day versus placebo. The cholestyramine group had a reduction in LDL-C of 12.6% greater than placebo. The cholestyramine group had a statistically significant 19% reduction in the primary endpoint of fatal CHD or nonfatal MI, with a 24% reduction in fatal CHD and 19% in nonfatal MI. This significant trial did support the use of cholestyramine in primary prevention patients to reduce the initial appearance of MI.

Colestipol has been studied in a small, difficult-to-interpret study of several thousand patients.[282] That study suggests event reduction with colestipol.

AGENTS AND DOSAGE

There are currently 3 bile acid-binding agents (or resins) on the market, cholestyramine and colestipol, both now generic, and colesevelam (Welchol). All 3 agents are now used primarily as add-on therapy for LDL-C lowering beyond that achievable with statin, and possibly in addition to ezetimibe therapy also.

The resins are all begun at a low initial dose and then titrated gradually until the target LDL-C is achieved, or side effects have become too prominent, or the maximum dose has been achieved. (See Table 22-1.)

Other Uses

Since these agents bind the bile salts in the intestine, they can be useful in reducing diarrhea in post-cholecystectomy patients who are having chronic diarrhea from the excess of bile salts in the intestine. Dosing is similar to that already discussed.

Since the agents are not absorbed systemically, they are the only cholesterol lowering agents that appear to be safe for use in the very rare fertile female who must have cholesterol lowering therapy, usually after referral to a lipid specialist.

SIDE EFFECTS

The side effect patterns of all these agents are similar. Since the agents are not absorbed but remain in the intestine, the side effects are all gastrointestinal in nature. These side effects include abdominal pain, abdominal distension, constipation, nausea, and vomiting. The side

Table 22-1 Dosage by Agent

Agent	Initial Dose	Maximum Dose
Cholestyramine	4 gm once or twice/day	24 gm twice daily
Colestipol	2 gm once or twice/day	15 gm twice daily
Colesevelam (Welchol)	1875 mg twice daily	7 tablets given (3 tablets BID) in divided doses[283–287]

effects appear to be very dose related, and they are frequently so significant that many patients are unable or unwilling to take one of these agents.

COMBINATION STUDIES WITH THE RESINS

The resin products were combined with niacin in several well known combination trials in the 1980s. The trials, CLAS-I, CLAS-II, and FATS, were angiographic trials and assessed whether aggressive cholesterol therapy could induce regression of atherosclerotic lesions already in existence in the coronary arteries. The trials detected that aggressive cholesterol lowering produced slowing of progression, or regression, of existing coronary lesions.[276,286,287]

Unfortunately, the trials were too small and too short to produce reduction in cardiac events. In our modern era, where we now recognize that plaque instability and plaque rupture are critical for cardiac events and disease progression, these trials, which presumed that the progression of atherosclerotic plaque was a slow and steady process, are of doubtful significance.

Chapter 23
Omega-3 Fish Oils

There has been an upsurge of interest, both on the part of practitioners and also patients, in the use of omega-3 fish oils. The evidence to support this enthusiasm is, in my opinion, quite lacking and heavily based on assumptions, so I present it carefully.

One of the stimulants for this interest is the observation that certain populations with diets heavy in fish and fish oils frequently have lower rates of cardiac events. There are huge problems with attempting to extrapolate for a certain specific treatment modality from population patterns. First is the fact that any population that eats a diet high in fish consumption will have much lower consumption of other foods (like cheeseburgers), frequently with less of the red meat and dairy that is a huge part of the Western diet. Secondly, these populations have many other differences with populations in the United States and Western Europe, namely dramatically different genetic risks, different rates of smoking, different rates of obesity and diabetes, and different levels of physical activity, all of which play a major part in determining the risks for cardiovascular disease. Thirdly, there frequently is an assumption that something that is "natural" like fish oil is inherently safe, since it is "natural." Nature is, of course, actually loaded with toxins, as organisms use these toxins to attack their foes. Many of these sources of toxins, like snake venom, have been adapted to provide medicinal compounds. However, "natural" does not necessarily mean "safe."

The current interest in the omega-3 fish oils is whether they are useful therapy in the management of patients with high cholesterol, particularly to lower triglycerides. Since there is no evidence that lowering triglycerides reduces cardiac events, I think significant caution should be maintained around this question.

EVIDENCE OF EFFICACY

The real interest in omega-3 oils came from a study published in 2002 in *Circulation*.[288] The study was a part of the GISSI program, and it evaluated 11,323 patients with a recent MI.

The patients were assigned omega-3 oils, vitamin E, both, or no treatment, in a randomized, but open-label (*not* placebo-controlled) trial. The patients who received the omega-3 oils had a significantly lower sudden cardiac death rate beginning within about 3 months, and this factor produced significant reductions in total mortality and cardiac mortality also, particularly early in the study. There was not a significant reduction in nonfatal MI, in spite of the mortality reductions. The mortality reduction did drive the primary endpoint (death, nonfatal MI, and nonfatal stroke) significantly down. The cholesterol values showed only minor changes, with the LDL-C essentially unchanged, along with the HDL-C. There was a very slight reduction (4.6%) in the triglycerides.

The authors noted that the majority of benefit was seen in the reduction of *sudden* cardiac death, and they concluded that the benefit from the omega-3 oils was as an anti-arrhythmic agent, not a cholesterol lowering agent.[288] Previous studies had also indicated that the agents manifested anti-arrhythmic properties.

Three follow-up studies are very important in understanding the effects of omega-3 agents. Because the benefit from omega-3 agents appeared to be through anti-arrhythmic properties, these studies evaluated their effects on patients with arrhythmic potential.[289–291] In the studies, patients with a previous history of ventricular arrhythmias and with implanted cardiac defibrillators were given omega-3 fish oils or placebo. None of the 3 studies showed a significant reduction in cardiac mortality or arrhythmias; indeed, 1 of the studies showed a trend for *increased* arrhythmias, consistent with the tendency for anti-arrhythmic agents also to be pro-arrhythmic.[291]

AGENTS AND DOSAGE

There is currently 1 prescription agent of omega-3-acid ethyl esters, marketed as Lovaza.[292] The preparation is dosed at 4 grams/day, taken either as four 1-gram capsules daily or two 1-gram capsules twice daily. It is approved for secondary use in addition to statin therapy for elevated triglycerides, or as monotherapy in patients with very high triglycerides (> 500 mg/dL). When it was added to simvastatin, it was shown to reduce triglycerides by an additional 23% with a 4.6% increase in HDL-C and no significant change in LDL-C.[292] When it was used as monotherapy in patients with very high triglycerides (> 500 mg/dL), it produced a 51% decrease in triglycerides but also produced a 49% *increase* in LDL-C.

RECOMMENDATIONS

At this point, I recommend that we do not use omega-3 fish oils. This recommendation is based on several key scientific points.

First, most practitioners presume that the treatment to lower triglycerides will reduce events. However, that has never been proven clinically, and, as I said in the triglyceride sections, I doubt that lowering triglycerides will reduce cardiovascular events. Therefore, there is no clear indication or consensus that such a treatment might be valuable.

Secondly, if the benefit in the GISSI trial was from anti-arrhythmic properties, as the authors concluded, the pro-arrhythmic potential seen in 1 of the defibrillator trials is ominous.[288,291] Should we use an unproven treatment that has suggested it might induce potentially lethal ventricular arrhythmias? With the potential for these very serious side effects and with no clearly proven clinical benefit (other than a laboratory test benefit of lowered triglycerides), I recommend we do not use this treatment. I would not take such an agent myself, and therefore I will not prescribe it for my patients.

Chapter 24

Torcetrapib

The story of torcetrapib is an extremely compelling account that clearly demonstrates how simply relying on improvements in cholesterol values without evidence for the reduction of cardiac events can be dangerous.

Briefly, torcetrapib was a CETP (cholesteryl ester transfer protein) inhibitor that dramatically raised the HDL-C level and also lowered LDL-C. There was tremendous interest in developing torcetrapib as a treatment to be added to statin therapy in a combination product.

Torcetrapib was studied in ILLUMINATE, a long-term trial enrolling more than 15,000 patients and randomizing them to atorvastatin with torcetrapib or to atorvastatin alone. The study was stopped after less than 2 years instead of the planned 5 years. In ILLUMINATE, torcetrapib did produce dramatic improvements in cholesterol values, raising HDL-C by 71% and lowering LDL-C by an additional 25%.

However, in this critical long-term trial, cardiovascular events were dramatically increased in the torcetrapib patients.[165] The study was terminated early because of a 25% increase in total mortality in the torcetrapib-treated patients, along with a 21% increase in fatal coronary disease, a 21% increase in nonfatal MI, and a 35% increase in hospitalizations for unstable angina in the torcetrapib patients. It was noted that the torcetrapib-treated patients had modest but definite increases in blood pressure, by 5 mm Hg systolic and 2 mm Hg diastolic pressures. Whether this 1 effect was potent enough to produce the increased cardiac events is not clear at this time.[293,294] Subsequent studies showed that torcetrapib did not slow the progression of atherosclerosis when it was measured by carotid B-mode ultrasonography and by coronary intravascular ultrasound.[295,296]

This failure of a potential therapy that was expected to offer dramatic improvements in cardiovascular treatment makes several important points. First, it emphasizes that we must have legitimate reductions in clinical events to know that a cholesterol treatment is truly successful, and that we cannot just rely on surrogate markers like laboratory values or measurements of atherosclerosis alone (without clinical events improvements) to determine whether treatments, particularly new treatments, are to be used.[297] Also, the benefit of adding secondary agents to raise HDL-C remains in question.[298] That question is, at least, unproven and in need of further study.

Chapter 25
Coenzyme Q_{10}

Coenzyme Q_{10} is a food supplement commonly used by the public and advocated by some practitioners for treatment of statin-related myalgia.

This treatment is very difficult to discuss in a publication like this, since there is almost no scientific information about whether it is at all safe or effective. Therefore, this discussion will be limited by the lack of clear information.

Statin myalgia is a symptomatic problem in which some users of statin therapy complain of diffuse muscle aches. One of the problems here is that there is no clear and well-recognized definition as to what statin myalgia really is.

Caution around this question is appropriate. With no clear laboratory tests or historical or physical findings, the proper diagnosis of statin myalgia is difficult. In fact, one of our greatest challenges is that patients frequently self-diagnose this condition and then present the issue to their practitioners.

I have several observations in attempting to assist you with this issue. First, statins are life-saving therapy, with success in reducing cardiovascular events across the complete spectrum of patients. Also, the safety of statins in these trials and in the general population is well-proven and genuine. Therefore, statins should not be casually stopped just because patients think they might have statin myalgia.

Secondly, the incidence of statin myalgia is probably vastly overstated. Some reports indicate that as many as 13.6% of patients report statin myopathy.[299] The recently completed JUPITER study found that 15.4% of the placebo patients and 16.0% of the rosuvastatin patients had myalgia, showing no difference between the placebo and statin patients, and also showing the same rate as reported earlier. The JUPITER study evaluated patients with a median age in the mid-60s. Therefore, we need to be careful not to overdiagnose the routine aches and pains of our advancing years as statin myalgia. The rates of myalgia in JUPITER suggest that statin myalgia is much less common than many of us assume.

Statin myalgia should have several features. Since it is a systemic issue, the muscle discomfort will be *bilateral*, affecting the muscle groups on both sides of the body equally. The clinical presentation is actually quite similar to polymyalgia rheumatica.

Statin myalgia is *not* joint pain. Joint pain is arthralgia, not myalgia, and arthralgia is not caused by statins. Also, there is usually a clear historical pattern to statin myalgia, usually starting within a few weeks of the onset of statin therapy. A specific clue to statin myalgia is that it sometimes appears with a statin dose escalation, say from 20 mg to 40 mg. Therefore, we need to begin the evaluation of a patient with possible statin myalgia by starting with a careful history about the onset of the symptoms, their location, and any new treatments or dose adjustments. Then, on physical exam, we should expect to detect some mild or more noticeable muscle tenderness, which should also be bilateral.

If we continue to suspect that the patient is suffering from statin myalgia, we should always check a CK level, which is normal if they have only myalgia instead of myopathy.

At this point, there again is no clear management consensus. My opinion is that statins are essential, life-saving therapy and that we therefore should make every effort to keep appropriate patients on a statin if possible. Also, as shown in Bryan Brewer's work (Figures 18-1 and 18-2), since the rate of myopathy is related to the milligram dose of the statin, not the LDL-C reduction, an excellent therapeutic option is to go to another, more potent statin. In myalgia patients who are on one of the older, less potent statins, we should take them off their original statin and wash them out for about 3 weeks. If they truly have statin myalgia, the myalgia should resolve in that time frame. Then we should rechallenge them with a very small dose of a more potent statin, usually rosuvastatin 5 mg. Since rosuvastatin is also somewhat hydrophilic, with less penetration of the muscles, most patients can tolerate this dose. If they do, frequently we can increase the dose gradually to achieve appropriate LDL-C control.

The coenzyme Q_{10} question is driven by a hypothesis that statin therapy may lead to mitochondrial dysfunction in muscle mitochondria by inhibiting the synthesis of coenzyme Q_{10}.[300] This hypothesis is just a "guess" as to what the cause of statin myalgia really is. Whether the supposed "depletion of muscle cell coenzyme Q_{10}" even occurs is unknown, so there is no scientific basis for assuming that this might be the cause of statin myalgia. Finally, whether oral supplementation of coenzyme Q_{10} could affect muscle cell coenzyme Q_{10} is also unknown. Therefore, the use of coenzyme Q_{10} is not supported by any scientific evidence.

EVIDENCE OF EFFICACY

There is no clear evidence that coenzyme Q_{10} has any efficacy beyond that of placebo. Since it is marketed as a "food supplement," the manufacturers need not prove the efficacy or safety of the coenzyme before marketing. Also, being a "supplement" means the manufacturers do not need scientific data to support their advertising claims.

There have been only 2 small pilot studies attempting to determine if coenzyme Q_{10} does reduce statin myalgia. Both studies are limited to being very small, brief pilot studies. They used pain scales to attempt to define the degree of myalgia pain. The better of the 2 studies used a double-blind, placebo-controlled format and studied 44 patients for 12 weeks. This study also used a controlled dose escalation schedule of simvastatin, to get consistent statin exposure for all the patients. This study found that coenzyme Q_{10} had no effect on statin myalgia symptoms.[299] The second study was smaller (only 32 patients), shorter (only 1 month), and used vitamin E instead of a placebo. This less scientific study did find a modest reduction in statin myalgia symptoms with coenzyme Q_{10}.[300]

At this point, there is no clear answer as to whether there is any value to coenzyme Q_{10} beyond placebo effect, which is certainly an important question in a pain symptom study.

RECOMMENDATION

At this point, there is no evidence beyond anecdotal support that coenzyme Q_{10} has any value. Also, we do not have any evidence that long-term administration of coenzyme Q_{10} is safe.

Because there is no scientific evidence that coenzyme Q_{10} is efficacious or safe, I do *not* recommend it to any of my patients, nor would I take it myself. I therefore urge you not to recommend it without more scientific documentation of its effectiveness or safety.

REFERENCES AND SUGGESTED READINGS

1. American Heart Association Statistics Committee and Stroke Statistics Subcommittee. Heart disease and stroke statistics–2008 update. *Circulation.* 2008;117:e25–e146.
2. Fox CS, Evans JC, Larson MG, Kannel WB, Levy D. Temporal trends in coronary heart disease mortality and sudden cardiac death from 1950 to 1999. *Circulation.* 2004;110:522–527.
3. Ford ES, Ajani UA, Croft JB, et al. Explaining the decrease in U.S. deaths from coronary disease, 1980–2000. *N Engl J Med.* 2007;356:2388–2398.
4. Goldman L, Phillips KA, Coxson P, et al. The effect of risk factor reductions between 1981 and 1990 on coronary heart disease incidence, prevalence, mortality and cost. *J Am Coll Cardiol.* 2001;38:1012–1017.
5. Laatikainen T, Critchley J, Vartianen E, Salomaa V, Ketonen M, Capewell S. Explaining the decline in coronary heart disease mortality in Finland between 1982 and 1997. *Amer J Epidemiol.* 2005;162: 764–773.
6. Hardoon SL, Whincup PH, Lennon LT, Wannamethee SG, Capewell S, Morris RW. How much of the recent decline in the incidence of myocardial infarction in British men can be explained by changes in cardiovascular risk factors? *Circulation.* 2008;117:598–604.
7. Luepker RV. Decline in incident coronary heart disease. Why are the rates falling? *Circulation.* 2008;117:592–593.
8. Nemetz PN, Roger VL, Ranson JE, Bailey KR, Edwards WD, Leibson CL. Recent trends in the prevalence of coronary disease. *Arch Intern Med.* 2008;166:264–270.
9. Olshansky SJ, Persky V. The canary in the coal mine. *Arch Intern Med.* 2008;168:261.
10. Veterans Administration Cooperative Study Group on Antihypertensive Agents. Effects of treatment on morbidity in hypertension. *JAMA.* 1967;202: 116–122.
11. Veterans Administration Cooperative Study Group on Antihypertensive Agents. Effects of treatment on morbidity in hypertension. II. Results in patients with diastolic blood pressure averaging 90 through 114 mm Hg. *JAMA.* 1970;213:1143–1152.
12. Collins R, Peto R, MacMahon S, et al. Blood pressure, stroke, and coronary heart disease. Part 2, short term reductions in blood pressure: overview of randomized drug trials in their epidemiological context. *Lancet.* 1990;335:827–838.
13. Vasan RS, Beiser A, Seshadri S, et al. Residual lifetime risk for developing hypertension in middle-aged women and men. *JAMA.* 2002;287:1003–1010.
14. SHEP Cooperative Research Group. Prevention of stroke by antihypertensive drug treatment in older persons with isolated systolic hypertension. *JAMA.* 1991;265:3255–3264.
15. Staessen JA, Thijs L, Celis H, et al. Randomised double-blind comparison of placebo and active treatment for older patients with isolated systolic hypertension. *Lancet.* 1997;350:757–764.
16. Insua JT, Sacks HS, Lau TS, et al. Drug treatment of hypertension in the elderly: a meta-analysis. *Ann Intern Med.* 1994;121:355–362.
17. Becket NS, Peters R, Fletcher AE, et al. Treatment of hypertension in patients 80 years of age or older. *N Engl J Med.* 2008;358:1887–1898.
18. Van den Hoogen PCW, Feskens EJM, Nagelkerke NJD, et al. The relation between blood pressure and mortality due to coronary heart disease among men in different parts of the world. *N Engl J Med.* 2000;342:1–8.
19. Ogden LG, He J, Lydick E, Whelton P. Long-term absolute benefit of lowering blood pressure in hypertensive patients according to the JNC VI risk stratification. *Hypertension.* 2000;35:539.
20. Burt VL, Whelton P, Rocella EJ, et al. Prevalence of hypertension in the US adult population. Results for the third National Health and Nutrition Examination Survey. *Hypertension.* 1995;25:305–313.
21. Hajjar H, Kotchen TA. Trends in prevalence, awareness, treatment, and control of hypertension in the United States, 1988–2000. *JAMA.* 2003;290:199–206.
22. Petrella RJ, Merikle EP, Jones J. Prevalence, treatment, and control of hypertension in primary care: gaps, trends, and opportunities. *J Clin Hypertens.* 2007;9:28–35.
23. The Sixth Report of the Joint National Committee of Prevention, Detection, Evaluation, and Treatment

of High Blood Pressure. *Arch Intern Med*.1997: 2413–2446.

24. Hansen TW, Kikuya M, Thijs L, et al. Diagnostic thresholds for ambulatory blood pressure moving lower: a review based on a meta-analysis—clinical implications. *J Clin Hypertens*. 2008;10:377–381.
25. Pickering T; American Society of Hypertension Ad Hoc Panel. Recommendations for the use of home (self) and ambulatory blood pressure monitoring. *Amer J Hypertens*. 1996;9:1–11.
26. Pickering T, White W. When and how to use self (home) and ambulatory blood pressure monitoring. *J Am Soc Hypertens*. 2008;2:119–124.
27. Treatment of Mild Hypertension Study Group. Treatment of mild hypertension study group final results. *JAMA*. 1993;270:713–724.
28. Farnett L, Mulrow CD, Linn WD, Lucey CR, Tuley MR. The J-curve phenomenon and the treatment of hypertension. *JAMA*. 1991;265:489–495.
29. Hansson L, Zanchetti A, Carruthers SG, et al. Effects of intensive blood pressure lowering and low-dose aspirin in patients with essential hypertension: principal results of the Hypertension Optimal Treatment randomised trial. *Lancet*. 1998;351:1755–1762.
30. Joint National Committee on the Prevention, Detection, Evaluation, and Treatment of High Blood Pressure. The JNC VII report. *JAMA*. 2003; 289:2560–2571.
31. Rosendorff C, Black HR, Cannon CP, et al. Treatment of hypertension in the prevention and management of ischemic heart disease: a scientific statement from the American Heart Association Council for High Blood Pressure Research and the Councils on Clinical Cardiology and Epidemiology and Prevention. *Circulation*. 2007;115:2761–2788.
32. Heart Failure Society of America. Managing patients with hypertension and heart failure. *J Card Fail*. 2006;12:e112–e114.
33. ALLHAT Officers and Coordinators for the ALLHAT Collaborative Research Group. Major outcomes in high-risk hypertensive patients randomized to angiotensin-converting enzyme inhibitor or calcium channel blocker vs diuretic. *JAMA*. 2002;288: 2981–2997.
34. Hansson L, Hedner T, Lund-Johansen P, et al. Randomised trial of the effects of calcium antagonists and beta-blockers on cardiovascular morbidity and mortality in hypertension: the Nordic Diltiazem (NORDIL) study. *Lancet*. 2000;356:359–365.
35. Brown MJ, Palmer CR, Castigne A, et al. Morbidity and mortality in patients randomised to double-blind treatment with a long-acting calcium-channel blocker or diuretic in the International Nifedipine GITS study: intervention as a goal in hypertension treatment (INSIGHT). *Lancet*. 2000;356:366–372.
36. Black HR, Elliott WJ, Grandits G, et al. Principal results of the controlled onset verapamil investigation of cardiovascular end points (CONVINCE) trial. *JAMA*. 2003;289:2073–2082.
37. Zanchetti A, Bond G, Hennig M, et al. Calcium antagonist lacidipine slows down progression of asymptomatic carotid atherosclerosis: principal results of the European Lacidipine Study on Atherosclerosis (ELSA), a randomized, double-blind, long-term trial. *Circulation*. 2002;106(19): 2422–2427.
38. Julius S, Kjeldsen SE, Weber M, et al. Outcomes in hypertensive patients at high cardiovascular risk treated with regimens based on valsartan or amlodipine: the VALUE trial. *Lancet*. 2004;363: 2022–2031.
39. Weber MA, Julius S, Kjeldsen SE, et al. Blood pressure dependent and independent effects of antihypertensive treatment on clinical events in the VALUE trial. *Lancet*. 2004;363:2049–2051.
40. Dahlof B, Sever PS, Poultzer NR, et al. Prevention of cardiovascular events with an antihypertensive regimen of amlodipine adding perindopril as required versus atenolol adding bendroflumethazide as required, in the Anglo-Scandinavian Cardiac Outcomes Trial-Blood Pressure Lowering Arm (ASCOT-BPLA): a multicentre randomised controlled trial. *Lancet*. 2005;366:895–906.
41. Wing LMH, Reid CM, Ryan P, et al. A comparison of outcomes with angiotensin-converting enzyme inhibitors and diuretics for hypertension in the elderly. *N Engl J Med*. 2003;348:583–592.
42. Jaqmerson K, Weber MA, Bakris GL, et al. Benazepril plus amlodipine or hydrochlorothiazide for hypertension in high-risk patients. *N Engl J Med*. 2008;359:2417–2428.
43. MERIT-HF Study Group. Effect of metoprolol CR/XL in chronic heart failure: Metoprolol CR/XL Randomised Intervention Trial in Congestive Heart Failure (MERIT-HF). *Lancet*. 1999;353:2001–2007.
44. Packer M, Coats AJS, Fowler MB, et al. Effect of carvedilol on survival in severe heart failure. *N Engl J Med*. 2001;344:1651–1658.

45. CIBIS-II Investigators and Committees. The Cardiac Insufficiency Bisoprolol Study II (CIBIS-II): a randomised trial. *Lancet*. 1999;353:9–13.
46. The Beta-Blocker Evaluation of Survival Trial Investigators. A trial of the beta-blocker bucindolol in patients with advanced chronic heart failure. *N Engl J Med*. 2001;344:1659–1667.
47. Poole-Wilson PA, Swedberg K, Cleland JGF, et al. Comparison of carvedilol and metoprolol on clinical outcomes in patients with chronic heart failure in the Carvedilol Or Metoprolol European Trial (COMET): randomised controlled trial. *Lancet*. 2003;362:7–13.
48. Materson BJ, Reda DJ, Cushman WC; Department of Veterans Affairs Cooperative Study Group on Antihypertensive Agents. Department of Veterans Affairs single-drug therapy of hypertension study. *Am J Hypertens*. 1995;8:189–192.
49. Bakris GL, Williams M, Dworkin L, et al. Preserving renal function in adults with hypertension and diabetes: a consensus approach. *Am J Kidney Dis*. 2000;36:646–661.
50. Tarazi RC, Dustan HP, Frohlich ED. Long-term thiazide therapy in essential hypertension: evidence for persistent alteration in plasma volume and rennin activity. *Circulation*. 1970;41:709–717.
51. Australian National Blood Pressure Study Management Committee. The Australian therapeutic trial in mild hypertension. *Lancet*. 1980;i:1261–1267.
52. Medical Research Council Working Party. MRC trial of treatment of mild hypertension: principal results. *BMJ*. 1985;291:97.
53. Dahlof B, Lindholm LH, Hansson L, Schersten B, Ekbom T, Wester PO. Morbidity and mortality in the Swedish trial in old people with hypertension (STOP-hypertension). *Lancet*. 1991;338: 1281–1286.
54. MRC Working Party. Medical Research Council trial of treatment of hypertension in older adults: principal results. *BMJ*. 1992;302:405–411.
55. Kochar M, Guthrie R, Triscari J, Kassler-Taub K, Reeves RA. Matrix study of irbesartan with hydrochlorothiazide in mild-to-moderate hypertension. *Am J Hypertens*. 1999;12:797–805.
56. Reisin E, Weir M, Falkner B, Hutchinson HG, Anzalone D, Tuck M; Treatment in Obese Patients with Hypertension (TROPHY) Study Group. Lisinopril versus hydrochlorothiazide in obese hypertensive patients. *Hypertension*. 1997;30:140–145.
57. Papademetriou V, Burris JF, Notargiacocmo A, Fletcher RD, Freis ED. Thiazide therapy is not a cause of arrhythmia in patients with systemic hypertension. *Arch Int Med*. 1988;148:1272–1276.
58. Grimm RH, Flack JM, Grandits GA, et al. Long-term effects on plasma lipids of diet and drugs to treat hypertension. *JAMA*. 1996;275:1549–1556.
59. Elliott WJ. Glucose and cholesterol elevations from diuretic therapy: intention to treat versus actual on-therapy experience. *Am J Hypertens*. 1993;6:1114.
60. CONSENSUS Study Group. Effects of enalapril on mortality in severe congestive heart failure. Results of the Cooperative North Scandinavia Enalapril Survival Study Group. *N Engl J Med*. 1987;316:1429.
61. Pfeffer MA, Braunwald E, Moye LA, et al. Effect of captopril on mortality in patients with left ventricular dysfunction after myocardial infarction. Results of the survival and ventricular enlargement trial: the SAVE investigators. *N Engl J Med*. 1992;327:669–677.
62. Kober L, Torp-Pedersen C, Carlsed J, et al. A clinical trial of the angiotensin-converting enzyme inhibitor trandolapril in patients with left ventricular dysfunction after myocardial infarction. *N Engl J Med*. 1995;333:1670–1676.
63. The SOLVD Investigators. Effect of enalapril on mortality and the development of heart failure in asymptomatic patients with reduced left ventricular ejection fractions. *N Engl J Med*. 1992;327: 685–691.
64. EUROPA Investigators. Efficacy of perindopril in reduction of cardiovascular events among patients with stable coronary artery disease: randomised, double-blind, placebo-controlled, multicentre trial (the EUROPA study). *Lancet*. 2003;362:782–788.
65. The Heart Outcomes Prevention Evaluation Study Investigators. Effects of angiotensin-converting enzyme inhibitor, ramipril, on cardiovascular events in high risk patients. *N Engl J Med*. 2000; 342:145–153.
66. PROGRESS Collaborative Group. Randomised trial of a perindopril-based blood-pressure-lowering regimen among 6105 individuals with previous stroke or transient ischaemic attack. *Lancet*. 2001;358:1033–1041.
67. Tatti P, Pahor M, Byingtaon RP, et al. Outcome results of the fosinopril versus amlodipine cardiovascular events randomized trial (FACET) in patients with hypertension and NIDDM. *Diabetes Care*. 1998;21(4):597–603.

68. Heart Outcomes Prevention Evaluation (HOPE) Study Investigators. Effects of ramipril on cardiovascular and microvascular outcomes in people with diabetes mellitus: results of the HOPE study and MICRO-HOPE substudy. *Lancet*. 2000;355:253–259.
69. Maschio G, Alberti D, Janin G, et al. Effect of the angiotensin-converting enzyme inhibitor benazepril on the progression of chronic renal insufficiency. *N Engl J Med*. 1996;334(15):939–945.
70. Lewis EJ, Hunsicker LG, Bain RP, Rhode RD; Collaborative Study Group. The effect of the angiotensin-converting enzyme inhibition on diabetic nephropathy. *N Engl J Med*. 1993;329:1456–1462.
71. The DREAM Trial Investigators. Effect of ramipril on the incidence of diabetes. *N Engl J Med*. 2006;355(15):1551–1562.
72. Schmeider RE, Martus P, Klingbell A. Reversal of left ventricular hypertrophy in essential hypertension: a meta-analysis of randomized double-blind studies. *JAMA*. 1996;275:1507–1513.
73. David D, Jallad N, Germino FW, et al. A comparison of the cough profile of fosinopril and enalapril in hypertensive patients with a history of ACE-inhibitor associated cough. *Am J Therapeut*. 1995;2:806–813.
74. Pahor M, Psaty BM, Alderman MH, et al. Health outcomes associated with calcium antagonists compared with other first-line antihypertensive therapies: a meta-analysis of randomised controlled trials. *Lancet*. 2000;356:1949–1954.
75. Stassen JA, Fagard RH, Birdenhager WH, et al; Systolic Hypertension in Europe (SYST-EUR) Trial Investigators. Calcium channel blockade and cardiovascular prognosis in the European Trial of Isolated Systolic Hypertension. *Hypertension*. 1998;32:410–416.
76. National Intervention Cooperative Study in Elderly Hypertensives Study Group. Randomized double-blind comparison of a calcium antagonist and a diuretic in elderly hypertensives. *Hypertension*. 1999;34:1129–1133.
77. Blood Pressure Lowering Treatment Trialists Collaboration. Effects of ACE inhibitors, calcium antagonists, and other blood-pressure-lowering drugs: results of prospectively designed overviews of randomised trials. *Lancet*. 2000;355:1955–1964.
78. Hanssonn L, Lindholm LH, Ekbornt T, et al. Randomised trial of old and new antihypertensive drugs in elderly patients: cardiovascular mortality and morbidity in the Swedish Trial in Old Patients with Hypertension-2 study. *Lancet*. 1999;354:1751–1756.
79. Black HR, Elliott WJ, Grandits G, et al. Principal results of the controlled onset verapamil investigation of cardiovascular end points (CONVINCE) trial. *JAMA*. 2003;289(16):2073–2082.
80. Rosei EA, Palu CD, Gastone L, et al; VHAS Investigators. Clinical results of the verapamil in hypertension atherosclerosis study. *J Hypertens*. 1997;15:1337–1344.
81. Estacio RO, Jeffers BW, Hiatt WR, et al. The effect of nislodipine as compared with enalapril on cardiovascular outcomes in patients with non-insulin-dependent diabetes and hypertension. *N Engl J Med*. 1998;338:645–652.
82. Agodoa LY, Appel L, Bakris GL, et al. Effect of ramipril vs amlodipine on renal outcomes in hypertensive nephrosclerosis. *JAMA*. 2001;285:2719–2728.
83. The Multicenter Diltiazem Postinfarction Trial Research Group. The effect of diltiazem on mortality and reinfarction after myocardial infarction. *N Engl J Med*. 1988;319:385–392.
84. Goldstein RE, Bocuzzi SJ, Cruess D, Nattel S. Diltiazem increases late-onset congestive heart failure in postinfarction patients with early reduction in ejection fraction. *Circulation*. 1991;83:52–60.
85. Francis GS. Calcium channel blockers and congestive heart failure. *Circulation*. 1991;83:336–338.
86. Littier WA, Sheridan DJ; UK Study Group. Placebo controlled trial of felodopine in patients with mild to moderate heart failure. *Br Heart J*. 1995;73:428–433.
87. Cohn JN, Ziesche S, Smith R, et al; Vasodilator-Heart Failure Trial (V-HeFT) Study Group. Effect of the calcium antagonist felodipine as supplementary vasodilator therapy in patients with chronic heart failure treated with enalapril: V-HeFT III. *Circulation*. 1997;96(3):856–863.
88. Packer M, O'Connor CM, Ghali J, et al; Prospective Amlodipine Survival Study Group. Effect of amlodipine on morbidity and mortality in severe chronic heart failure. *N Engl J Med*. 1996;335(15):1107–1114.
89. Pitt B, Byington RP, Furberg CD, et al; PREVENT Investigators. Effect of amlodipine on the progression of atherosclerosis and the occurrence of clinical events. *Circulation*. 2000;102:1503–1510.
90. Kassler-Taub K, Littlejohn T, Elliott W, Ruddy T, Adler E; Irbesartan/Losartan Study Investigators.

Comparative efficacy of two angiotensin II receptor antagonists, irbesartan and losartan, in mild-to-moderate hypertension. *Am J Hypertens*. 1998;11:445–453.

91. Oparil S, Guthrie R, Lewin AJ, et al; Irbesartan Losartan Study Investigators. An elective titration study of the comparative effectiveness of two angiotensin II receptor blockers, irbesartan and losartan. *Clin Therapeut*. 1998;20:398–409.
92. Atacand [package insert]. Wilmington, DE: AstraZeneca LP; 2007.
93. White WB, Lacourciere Y, Davidai G. Effects of the angiotensin II receptor blockers telmisartan versus valsartan on the circadian variation of blood pressure. *Am J Hypertens*. 2004;17:347–353.
94. White WB, Punzi HA, Murwin D, Koval SE, Davidai G, Neutel JM. Effects of the angiotensin II receptor blockers telmisartan vs. valsartan in combination with hydrochlorothiazide 25 mg once daily for the treatment of hypertension. *J Clin Hypertens*. 2006;8:626–633.
95. White WB, Murwin D, Chrysant SG, Koval SE, Davidai, Guthrie R. Effects of the angiotensin II receptor blockers telmisartan versus valsartan in combination with hydrochlorothiazide: a large, confirmatory trial. *Blood Press Monit*. 2008; 13:21–27.
96. Oparil S, Williams D, Chrysant SG, Marbury TC, Neutel J. Comparative efficacy of olmesartan, losartan, valsartan, and irbesartan in the control of essential hypertension. *J Clin Hypertens*. 2001;3:283–292.
97. Dahlof B, Defvereux RB, Kjeldsen SE, et al; LIFE Study Group. Cardiovascular morbidity and mortality in the Losartan Intervention For Endpoint reduction in hypertension study (LIFE): a randomised trial against atenolol. *Lancet*. 2002;359:995–1003.
98. Dicksteinn K, Kjekhus J; OPTIMAAL Steering Committee. Effects of losartan and captopril on mortality and morbidity in high-risk patients after acute myocardial infarction: the OPTIMAAL randomised trial. *Lancet*. 2002;360:752–760.
99. Pfeffer MA, McMurray JJV, Velazquez EJ, et al. Valsartan, captopril or both in myocardial infarction complicated by heart failure, left ventricular dysfunction, or both. *N Engl J Med*. 2003;349: 1893–1906.
100. Pitt B, Segal R, Martinez FA, et al. Randomised trial of losartan versus captopril in patients over 65 with heart failure (Evaluation of Losartan in the Elderly Study, ELITE). *Lancet*. 1997;349:747–752.
101. Pitt B, Poole-Wilson PA, Segal R, et al. Effect of losartan compared with captopril on mortality in patients with symptomatic heart failure: randomised trial—the Losartan Heart Failure Survival Study ELITE II. *Lancet*. 2000;355:1582–1587.
102. Cohn JN, Tognoni G; Valsartan Heart Failure Trial Investigators. A randomised trial of the angiotensin-receptor blocker valsartan in chronic heart failure. *N Engl J Med*. 2001;345:1667–1675.
103. Pfeffer MA, Swedberg K, Granger CB, et al. Effects of candesartan on mortality and morbidity in patients with chronic heart failure: the CHARM-Overall program. *Lancet*. 2003;362:759–766.
104. McMurray JJV, Ostergren J, Swedberg K, et al. Effects of candesartan in patients with chronic heart failure and reduced left-ventricular systolic function taking angiotensin-converting enzyme inhibitors: the CHARM-Added trial. *Lancet*. 2003; 362:767–771.
105. Granger CB, McMurray JJV, Yusuf S, et al. Effects of candesartan in patients with chronic heart failure and reduced left-ventricular systolic intolerant to angiotensin-converting enzyme inhibitors: the CHARM-Alternative trial. *Lancet*. 2003;362: 772–776.
106. Yusuf S, Pfeffer MA, Swedberg K, et al. Effects of candesartan in patients with chronic heart failure and preserved left-ventricular ejection fraction: the CHARM Preserved trial. *Lancet*. 2003;362:777–781.
107. The ONTARGET Investigators. Telmisartan, ramipril, or both in patients at high risk for vascular events. *N Engl J Med*. 2008;358:1547–1559.
108. Telmisartan Randomised Assessment Study in ACE intolerant subjects with Cardiovascular Disease (TRANSCEND) Investigators. Effects of the angiotensin-receptor blocker telmisartan on cardiovascular events in high-risk patients intolerant to angiotensin-converting enzyme inhibitors: a randomised controlled trial. *Lancet*. 2008;372: 1174–1183.
109. Brenner BM, Cooper ME, DeZeeuw D, et al. Effects of losartan on renal and cardiovascular outcomes in patients with Type 2 diabetes and nephropathy. *N Engl J Med*. 2001;345:861–869.
110. Parving HH, Lenhart H, Brochner, Mortensen J, et al. The effect of irbesartan on the development of diabetic nephropathy in patients with Type 2 diabetes. *N Engl J Med*. 2001;345:870–878.
111. Lewis EJ, Hunsicker LG, Clarke WR, et al. Renoprotective effect of the angiotensin-receptor antagonist irbesartan in patients with nephropathy

due to Type 2 diabetes. *N Engl J Med*. 2001;345: 851–860.

112. Hilgers KF, Mann JFE. ACE Inhibitors versus AT1 receptor antagonists in patients with chronic renal disease. *J Am Soc Nephrol*. 2002;13: 1100–1108.
113. Man JFE, Schmieder RE, McQueen MM, et al. Renal outcomes with telmisartan, ramipril, or both in patients at high vascular risk (the ONTARGET study): a multicentre, randomised, double-blind, controlled trial. *Lancet*. 2008;372:547–553.
114. Wilhemsen L, Berglund G, Elmfeldt D, et al. Beta-blockers versus diuretics in hypertensive men: main results from the HAPPHY trial. *J Hypertens*. 1987;5:561–572.
115. Wikstrand J, Warnold I, Tuomilehto J, et al. Metoprolol versus thiazide diuretics in hypertension. Morbidity results from the MAPHY Study. *Hypertension*. 1991;17:579–588.
116. Messerli FH, Grossman E, Goldbourt U. Are beta-blockers efficacious as first-line therapy for hypertension in the elderly? *JAMA*. 1998;279:1903–1907.
117. Bangalore S, Parkar S, Grossman E, Messeerli FH. A meta-analysis of 94,492 patients with hypertension treated with beta blockers to determine the risk of new-onset diabetes mellitus. *Am J Cardiol*. 2007;100:1254–1263.
118. Timolol-induced reduction in mortality and reinfarction in patients surviving acute myocardial infarction. *N Engl J Med*. 1981;304:801–807.
119. A randomized trial of propranolol in patients with acute myocardial infarction. I. Mortality results. *JAMA*. 1982;247:1707–1714.
120. Kasiske BL, Ma JZ, Kalil RSN, Louis TA. Effects of antihypertensive therapy on serum lipids. *Ann Intern Med*. 1995;122:133–141.
121. The Antihypertensive and Lipid-Lowering Treatment to Prevent Heart Attack Trial (ALLHAT). Major cardiovascular events in hypertensive patients randomized to doxazosin vs. chlorthalidone. *JAMA*. 2000;283:1967–1975.
122. Chapman N, Chang CL, Dahlof B, et al. Effect of doxazosin gastrointestinal therapeutic system as third line antihypertensive therapy on blood pressure and lipids in the Anglo-Scandinavian Outcomes Trial. *Circulation*. 2008;118:42–48.
123. Guthrie R. Terazosin in the treatment of hypertension and symptomatic benign prostatic hyperplasia: a primary care trial. *J Fam Pract*. 1994;39: 129–133.
124. Guthrie RM, Siegel RM; Hypertension and BPH Intervention (HABIT) Multicenter Study Group. A multi-center, community-based study of doxazosin in the treatment of concomitant hypertension and symptomatic benign prostatic hyperplasia: the Hypertension and BPH Intervention Trial. *Clin Therapeut*. 1999;21:1732–1747.
125. Tekturna [package insert]. East Hanover, NJ: Novartis Pharmaceuticals; 2007.
126. Pitt B, Remme W, Zannad F, et al. Eplerenone, a selective aldosterone blocker, in patients with left ventricular dysfunction after myocardial infarction. *N Engl J Med*. 2003;348:1309–1321.
127. Inspra [package insert]. New York: G.D. Searle LLC; 2008.
128. Conn JN, Archibald DG, Ziesche S, et al. Effect of vasodilator therapy on mortality in chronic congestive heart failure. Results of a Veterans Administration Cooperative Study. *N Engl J Med*. 1982;314:1547–1552.
129. Taylor AL, Ziesche S, Yancy C, et al. Combination of isosorbide and hydralazine in blacks with heart failure. *N Engl J Med*. 2004;351:2049–2057.
130. Coronary Drug Project Research Group. Clofibrate and niacin in coronary heart disease. *JAMA*. 1975; 231:360–381.
131. Committee of Principal Investigators. A co-operative trial in the primary prevention of ischaemic heart disease using clofibrate. *Br Heart J*. 1978;40: 1069–1118.
132. The Lipid Research Clinics Program. The Lipids Research Clinics Coronary Primary Prevention Trial results. *JAMA*. 1984;251:351–364.
133. Frick MH, Elo O, Happa K, et al. Helsinki Heart Study: primary-prevention trial with gemfibrozil in middle-aged men with dyslipidemia. *N Engl J Med*. 1987;317:1237–1245.
134. Steinberg D. The statins in primary prevention. *N Engl J Med*. 2008;359:1426–1427.
135. Lloyd-Jones DM, Larson MG, Beisler A, Levy D. Lifetime risk of developing coronary heart disease. *Lancet*. 1999;353:89–92.
136. Expert Panel on Detection, Evaluation, and Treatment of High Blood Cholesterol in Adults. Executive summary of the Third Report on the National Cholesterol Education Program (NCEP) expert panel on detection, evaluation, and treatment of high blood pressure in adults (Adult Treatment Panel III). *JAMA*. 2001;285:2486–2497.
137. Stamler J, Wentworth D, Neaton JD. Is relationship between serum cholesterol and risk of premature

death from coronary heart disease continuous and graded? Findings in 356,222 primary screenees of the Multiple Risk Factor Intervention Trial (MRFIT). *JAMA*. 1986;256:2823–2828.

138. Anderson KM, Castelli WP, Levy D. Cholesterol and mortality. 30 years of follow up from the Framingham Study. *JAMA*. 1987;257:2126–2180.
139. Castelli WP, Garrison RJ, Wilson PW, Abbott RD, Kalousdian S, Kannel WB. Incidence of coronary heart disease and lipoprotein levels. The Framingham Study. *JAMA*. 1986;256:2835–2838.
140. Kronmal RA, Cain KC, Ye Z, Omenn GS. Total serum cholesterol levels and mortality risk as a function of age. *Arch Intern Med*. 1993;153: 1065–1073.
141. Wong ND, Wilson PWF, Kannel WB. Serum cholesterol as a prognostic factor after myocardial infarction: The Framingham Study. *Ann Intern Med*. 1991;115:687–693.
142. Lloyd-Jones DM, Leip EP, Larson MG, et al. Prediction of lifetime risk for cardiovascular disease by a risk factor burden at 50 years of age. *Circulation*. 2006;113:791–798.
143. Pekkanen J, Heiss G, Suchindran CM, Leon A, Rifkind BM, Tyroler HA. Ten-year mortality from cardiovascular disease in relation to cholesterol level among men with and without preexisting cardiovascular disease. *N Engl J Med*. 1990;322:1700–1707.
144. Stamler J, Daviglus ML, Garside DB, et al. Relationship of baseline serum cholesterol in 3 large cohorts of younger men to long-term coronary, cardiovascular, and all-cause mortality and to longevity. *JAMA*. 2000;284:311–318.
145. Law MR, Wald NJ, Hackshaw A, Bailey A. Systematic underestimation of association between serum cholesterol concentration and ischaemic heart disease in observational studies: data from the BUPA study. *BMJ*. 1994;308:363–366.
146. Wilson PWF, D'Agostino R, Levy D, et al. Prediction of coronary heart disease using risk factor categories. *Circulation*. 1998;97:1837–1847.
147. Carroll MD, Lacher DA, Sorlie PD, et al. Trends in serum lipids and lipoproteins of adults, 1960–2002. *JAMA*. 2005;294:1773–1781.
148. The Women's Health Initiative Randomized Controlled Dietary Modification Trial. Low-fat dietary pattern and risk of cardiovascular disease. *JAMA*. 2006;295:655–666.
149. Grundy SM, Cleeman JI, Merz NB, et al. Implications of recent clinical trials for the National Cholesterol Education Program Adult Treatment Panel III Guidelines. *Circulation*. 2004;110:227–239.
150. Crouse JR, Raichlen JS, Riley WA, et al. Effect of rosuvastatin on progression of carotid intima-media thickness in low-risk individuals with subclinical atherosclerosis. The METEOR Trial. *JAMA*. 2007;297:1344–1353.
151. Nissen SE, Tuzcu EM, Schoenhagen P, et al. Effect of intensive compared with moderate lipid-lowering on therapy on progression of coronary atherosclerosis. *JAMA*. 2004;291:1071–1080.
152. Howard BV, Roman MJ, Devereux RB, et al. Effect of lower targets for randomized trial. *JAMA*. 2008;299:1678–1689.
153. Nissen SE, Nicholls SJ, Sipahi I, et al. Effect of very high-intensity statin therapy on regression of coronary atherosclerosis. The ASTEROID Trial. *JAMA*. 2006;295(13):1556–1565.
154. Ridker PM, Danielson E, Fonseca FAH, et al. Rosuvastatin to prevent vascular events in men and women with elevated C-reactive protein. *N Engl J Med*. 2008;359:2195–2207.
155. Corti MC, Guarainik JM, Salive ME, et al. HDL Cholesterol predicts coronary heart disease mortality in older persons. *JAMA*. 1995;274:539–544.
156. Barter P, Gotto AM, LaRosa JC, et al. HDL cholesterol, very low levels of LDL cholesterol, and cardiovascular events. *N Engl J Med*. 2007;357:1301–1310.
157. Wolfram RM, Brewer BB, Xue Z, et al. Impact of low high-density lipoproteins on in-hospital events and one year clinical outcomes in patients with non-ST-elevation myocardial infarction acute coronary syndrome treated with drug-eluting stent implantation. *Am J Cardiol*. 2006;98:711–717.
158. Guthrie RM. How safe is aggressive statin therapy? *Progress Cardiovasc Nurs*. 2006;21(3):140–144.
159. Manninen V, Elo MO, Frick MH, et al. Lipid alterations and decline in the incidence of coronary heart disease in the Helsinki Heart Study. *JAMA*. 1988;260:641–651.
160. Rubins HB, Robins SJ, Collins D, et al; Veterans Affairs High-Density Lipoprotein Cholesterol Intervention Trial Study Group. Gemfibrozil for the secondary prevention of coronary heart disease in men with low levels of high-density lipoprotein cholesterol. *N Engl J Med*. 1999;341(6):410–418.
161. Robins SJ, Collins D, Wittes JT; VA-HIT Study Group. Relation of gemfibrozil treatment and lipid levels with major coronary events. *JAMA*. 2001;285:1585–1591.

162. Downs JR, Clearfield M, Weis S, et al. Primary prevention of acute coronary events with lovastatin in men and women with average cholesterol. Results of AFCAPS/TexCAPS. *JAMA*. 1998;279(20): 1615–1622.
163. Gotto AM, Whitney E, Stein EA, et al. Relation between baseline and on-treatment lipid parameters and first acute major coronary events in the Air Force/Texas Coronary Atherosclerosis Prevention Study (AFCAPS/TexCAPS). *Circulation*. 2000;101:477–484.
164. VanderSteeg WA, Holme I, Boekholdt SM, et al. High-density lipoprotein cholesterol, high-density lipoprotein particle size, and apolipoprotein A-1: significance for cardiovascular risk. The IDEAL and Norfolk studies. *J Am Coll Cardiol*. 2008;51:634–642.
165. Barter PJ, Caulfield M, Eriksson M, et al. Effects of torcetrapib in patients at high risk for coronary events. *N Engl J Med*. 2007;357:2109–2122.
166. Genest J. The yin and yang of high-density lipoprotein cholesterol. *J Am Coll Cardiol*. 2008;51:643–644.
167. Nordestgaard BG, Benn M, Schnohr P, Tybjaerg-Hansen A. Nonfasting triglycerides and risk of myocardial infarction, ischemic heart disease, and death in men and women. *JAMA*. 2007;298:299–308.
168. Haim M, Benderly M, Brunner D, et al. Elevated serum triglyceride levels and long-term mortality in patients with coronary heart disease. The Benzafibrate Infarction Prevention (BIP) Registry. *Circulation*. 1999;100(5):475–482.
169. Sarwar N, Danesh J, Eriksurdsson G, et al. Triglycerides and the risk of coronary heart disease. *Circulation*. 2007;115:450–458.
170. Brunzell JD. Hypertriglyceridemia. *N Engl J Med*. 2007;357:1009–1017.
171. West of Scotland Coronary Prevention Study Group. Influence of pravastatin and plasma lipids on clinical events in the West of Scotland Coronary Prevention Study (WOSCOPS). *Circulation*. 1998;97:1440–1445.
172. Pedersen TR, Olsson AG, Faergeman O, et al. Lipoprotein changes and reduction in the incidence of major coronary heart disease events in the Scandinavian Simvastatin Survival Study (4S). *Circulation*. 1998;97:1453–1460.
173. O'Riordan M. IDEAL: Lowering triglycerides in stable statin-treated CHD patients does not provide benefit. *Heartwire*. May 2, 2008. http://www.theheart.org/article/861533.do. Accessed January 22, 2009.
174. Miller M, Cannon CP, Murphy SA, Qin J, Ray KK, Braunwald E. Impact of triglyceride levels beyond low-density lipoprotein cholesterol after acute coronary syndrome in the PROVE IT-TIMI 22 Trial. *J Am Coll Cardiol*. 2008;51:724–730.
175. Cui Y, Blumenthal RS, Flaws JA, et al. Non-high-density lipoprotein cholesterol level as a predictor of cardiovascular disease mortality. *Arch Intern Med*. 2001;161:1413–1419.
176. Grundy SM. Non-high-density lipoprotein cholesterol level as potential risk predictor and target therapy. *Arch Intern Med*. 2001;161:1379–1380.
177. Sniderman AD, Furberg CD, Keech A, et al. Apolipoproteins versus lipids as indices of coronary risk and as targets for statin treatment. *Lancet*. 2003;361:777–780.
178. Pischon T, Girman CJ, Sacks FM, Rifai N, Stampfer MJ, Rimm EB. Non-high-density lipoprotein cholesterol and apolipoprotein B in the prediction of coronary heart disease in men. *Circulation*. 2005;112:3375–3383.
179. Sattar N, Williams K, Sniderman AD, D'Agostino R, Haffner S. Comparison of the associations of apolipoprotein B and non-high-density lipoprotein cholesterol with other cardiovascular risk factors in patients with the metabolic syndrome. *Circulation*. 2004;110: 2687–2693.
180. Sniderman AD. Apolipoprotein B versus non-high-density lipoprotein cholesterol. *Circulation*. 2005;112:3366–3367.
181. Ridker PM, Stampfer MJ, Rifai N. Novel risk factors for systemic atherosclerosis. *JAMA*. 2001;285: 2481–2485.
182. Ebbing M, Bleie O, Ueland PM, et al. Mortality and cardiovascular events in patients treated with homocysteine-lowering B vitamins after coronary angiography. *JAMA*. 2008;300(7):795–804.
183. Ridker PM, Rifai N, Rose L, Buring JE, Cook NR. Comparison of C-reactive protein and low-density lipoprotein cholesterol levels in the prediction of first cardiovascular events. *N Engl J Med*. 2002;347:1557–1565.
184. Danesh J, Wheeler JG, Hirschfield BM, et al. C-reactive protein and other circulating markers of inflammation in the prediction of coronary heart disease. *N Engl J Med*. 2004;350:1387–1397.
185. Harris TB, Ferrucci L, Tracy RP, et al. Associations of elevated interleukin-6 and C-reactive protein levels with mortality in the elderly. *Am J Med*. 1999;106:506–512.

186. Tice JA, Browner W, Tracy RP, Cummings SR. The relation of C-reactive protein levels to total and cardiovascular mortality in older US women. *Am J Med*. 2003;114:199–205.
187. Cushman M, Arnold AM, Psaty BM, et al. C-reactive protein and the 10-year incidence of coronary heart disease in older men and women: The Cardiovascular Health Study. *Circulation*. 2005;112:25–31.
188. Wang TJ, Gona P, Larson MG, et al. Multiple biomarkers for the prediction of first major cardiovascular events and death. *N Engl J Med*. 2006;355:2631–2639.
189. Folsom AA, Chambless LE, Ballantyne CM, et al. An assessment of incremental coronary risk prediction using C-reactive protein and other novel risk markers. *Arch Intern Med*. 2006;166:1368–1373.
190. Wilson PWF, Nam BH, Pencina M, D'Agostino RB, Benjamin EJ, O'Donnell CJ. C-reactive protein and risk of cardiovascular disease in men and women from the Framingham Heart Study. *Arch Intern Med*. 2005;165:2473–2478.
191. Ridker PM, Buring JE, Cook NR, Rifai N. C-reactive protein, the metabolic syndrome, and risk of incident cardiovascular events: an 8-year follow-up of 14,719 initially healthy American women. *Circulation*. 2003;107:391–397.
192. Ridker PM, Wilson PWF, Grundy SM. Should C-reactive protein be added to metabolic syndrome and to assessment of global cardiovascular risk? *Circulation*. 2004;109:2818–2825.
193. Yeh ETH, Willerson JT. Coming of age of C-reactive protein: using inflammatory markers in cardiology. *Circulation*. 2003;107:370–371.
194. Zacho J, Tybjaerg-Hansen A, Jensen JS, Grande P, Sillesen H, Nordestgaard BG. Genetically elevated C-reactive protein and ischemic vascular disease. *N Engl J Med*. 2008;359:1897–1908.
195. Schunkert H, Samani NJ. Elevated C-reactive protein in atherosclerosis—chicken or egg? *N Engl J Med*. 2008;359:1953–1955.
196. Pearson TA, Mensah GA, Alexander RW, et al. Markers of inflammation and cardiovascular disease: application to clinical and public health practice: a statement from the Centers for Disease Control and Prevention and the American Heart Association. *Circulation*. 2003;107:499–511.
197. Ridker PM. Clinical application of C-reactive protein for cardiovascular disease detection and prevention. *Circulation*. 2003;107:363–369.
198. Grundy SM, Cleeman JI, Daniels SR, et al. Diagnosis and management of the metabolic syndrome: an American Heart Association/National Heart, Lung, and Blood Institute Executive Summary. *Circulation*. 2005;112:2735–2752.
199. American Diabetes Association. Metabolic syndrome: "Metabolic syndrome: a misleading diagnosis." News Release. August 25, 2005. http://www.diabetesmonitor.com/pr41.htm. Accessed January 22, 2009.
200. US Preventive Services Task Force. US Department of Health and Human Services, Agency for Healthcare Research and Quality. Screening for Coronary Heart Disease. February 2004. http://www.ahrq.gov/clinic/uspstf/uspsacad.htm. Accessed January 22, 2009.
201. Rank B. Executive physicals—bad medicine on three counts. *N Engl J Med*. 2008;359:1424–1425.
202. Greenland P, Bonow RO, Brundage BH, et al. ACCF/AHA 2007 clinical expert consensus document on coronary artery calcium scoring by computed tomography in global cardiovascular risk assessment and in evaluation of patients with chest pain. *Circulation*. 2007;115:402–426.
203. Arad Y, Spadaro LA, Roth M, Newstein D, Guerci AD. Treatment of asymptomatic adults with coronary calcium scores with atorvastatin, vitamin C, and vitamin E. *J Am Coll Cardiol*. 2005;46:166–172.
204. Raggi P, Davidson M, Callister TQ, et al. Aggressive versus moderate lipid-lowering therapy in hypercholesterolemic postmenopausal women: Beyond Endorsed Lipid Lowering With EBT Scanning (BELLES). *Circulation*. 2005;112:563–571.
205. Steinberg D. The statins in preventive cardiology. *N Engl J Med*. 2008;359:1426–1427.
206. Corsini A, Ferri N, Cortellaro M. Are pleiotropic effects of statins real? *Vasc Health Risk Manag*. 2007;3:1–3.
207. Scandinavian Simvastatin Survival Study Group. Randomized trial of cholesterol lowering in 4444 patients with coronary heart disease: the Scandinavian Simvastatin Survival Study (4S). *Lancet*. 1994;344:1383–1389.
208. The Long-Term Intervention with Pravastatin in Ischaemic Disease (LIPID) Study Group. Prevention of cardiovascular events and death with pravastatin in patients with coronary heart disease and a broad range of initial cholesterol levels. *N Engl J Med*. 1998;339:1349–1357.

209. Sachs FM, Pfeffer MA, Moye LA, et al. The effect of pravastatin on coronary events after myocardial infarction in patients with average cholesterol levels. *N Engl J Med*. 1996;335:1001–1009.
210. Serruys PW, deFeyter P, Macaya C, et al. Fluvastatin for prevention of cardiac events following successful first percutaneous coronary intervention. *JAMA*. 2002;287:3215–3222.
211. Spencer FA, Allegrone J, Goldberg RJ, et al. Association of statin therapy with outcomes of acute coronary syndromes: the GRACE Study. *Ann Intern Med*. 2004;140:857–866.
212. Heart Protection Study Collaborative Group. MRC/BHF Heart Protection Study of cholesterol lowering with simvastatin in 20,536 high-risk individuals: a randomized placebo-controlled trial. *Lancet*. 2002;360:7–22.
213. Shepherd J, Cobbe SM, Ford I, et al. Prevention of coronary heart disease with pravastatin in men with hypercholesterolemia. *N Engl J Med*. 1995;333:1301–1307.
214. Ford I, Murray H, Packard CJ, et al. Long-term follow-up of the West of Scotland Coronary Prevention Study. *N Engl J Med*. 2007;357:1477–1486.
215. Shepherd J, Blauw GJ, Murphy MB, et al. Pravastatin in elderly patients at risk of vascular disease (PROSPER): a randomised controlled trial. *Lancet*. 2002;360:1623–1630.
216. Sever PS, Dahlof B, Poulter NR, et al. Prevention of coronary and stroke events with atorvastatin in hypertensive patients who have average or lower-than-average cholesterol concentrations, in the Anglo-Scandinavian Cardiac Outcomes Trial-Lipid Lowering Arm (ASCOT-LLA): a multicenter randomised controlled trial. *Lancet*. 2003;361:1149–1157.
217. The ALLHAT Officers and Coordinators for the ALLHAT Collaborative Research Group. Major outcomes in moderately hypercholesterolemic, hypertensive patients randomized to pravastatin vs. usual care. *JAMA*. 2002;288:2998–3007.
218. Pasternak RC. The ALLHAT lipid lowering trial—less is less. *JAMA*. 2002;288:3042–3044.
219. Mizuno K, Nakaya N, Ohashi Y, et al. Usefulness of pravastatin in primary prevention of cardiovascular events in women. *Circulation*. 2008;117:494–502.
220. Calhoun HM, Betteridge DJ, Hitman G, et al. Primary prevention of cardiovascular disease with atorvastatin in type 2 diabetes in the Collaborative Atorvastatin Diabetes Study (CARDS): multicentre randomised placebo-controlled trial. *Lancet*. 2004;364:685–696.
221. Cannon CP, Braunwald E, McCabe CH, et al. Intensive versus moderate lipid lowering with statins after acute coronary syndromes. *N Engl J Med*. 2004;350:1495–1504.
222. LaRosa JC, Grundy SM, Waters DD, et al. Intensive lipid lowering with atorvastatin in patients with stable coronary disease. *N Engl J Med*. 2005;352:1425–1435.
223. Pedersen TR, Faergeman O, Kastelein JJ, et al. High-dose atorvastatin vs. usual-dose simvastatin for secondary prevention after myocardial infarction. The IDEAL Study. *JAMA*. 2005;294:2437–2445.
224. DeLemos JA, Blazing MA, Wiviott SD, et al. Early intensive vs. a delayed conservative simvastatin strategy in patients with acute coronary syndromes. *JAMA*. 2004;292:1307–1316.
225. Mevacor [package insert]. Whitehouse Station, NJ: Merck and Company; 2007.
226. Jones PH, Davidson MH, Stein EA, et al. Comparison of the efficacy and safety of rosuvastatin versus atorvastatin, simvastatin, and pravastatin across doses (STELLAR Trial). *Am J Cardiol*. 2003;92:152–160.
227. Zocor [package insert]. Whitehouse Station, NJ: Merck and Company; 2007.
228. Lescol [package insert]. East Hanover, NJ: Novartis Pharmaceuticals; 2006.
229. Lipitor [package insert]. Morris Plains, NJ: Parke-Davis; 2007.
230. Crestor [package insert]. Wilmington, DE: AstraZeneca; 2007.
231. White MC. HMG CoA reductase inhibitor-induced muscle toxicity: risks, monitoring, and management. *Formulary*. 2002;37:588–593.
232. Brewer HB. Benefit-risk assessment of rosuvastatin 10 to 40 milligrams. *Am J Cardiol*. 2003;92(supp):23K–29K.
233. Evans M. Statin safety in perspective—maximizing the risk:benefit. *Br J Cardiol*. 2004;11:449–454.
234. Downs JR, Clearfield M, Tyroler HA, et al. (Air Forse/Texas Coronary Atherosclerosis Prevention Study 9AFCAPS/TexCAPS): additional perspectives on tolerability of long-term treatment with lovastatin. *Am J Cardiol*. 2001;87:1074–1079.
235. Jacobson T. Statin safety: lessons from new drug applications for marketed statins. *Am J Cardiol*. 2006;97(suppl):44C–51C.

236. deDenus S, Spinler SA, Miller D, Peterson AM. Statins and liver toxicity: a meta-analysis. *Pharmacotherapy*. 2004;24:584–591.
237. Bays H. Ezetimibe. *Expert Opin Investig Drugs*. 2002;11:1587–1604.
238. Tolman KG. Defining patient risks from extended preventive therapies. *Am J Cardiol*. 2000;85:15E–19E.
239. Russo MW, Galanko JA, Shrestha R, Fried MW, Watkins P. Liver transplantation for acute liver failure from drug induced liver injury in the United States. *Liver Transpl*. 2004;10:1018–1023.
240. Dujovne CA. Side effects of statins: hepatitis versus "transaminitis"—myositis versus "CPKitis." *Am J Cardiol*. 2002;89:1411–1413.
241. Chituri S, George J. Hepatotoxicity of commonly used drugs: non-steroidal antiinflammatory drugs, antihypertensives, antidiabetic drugs, anticonvulsants, lipid-lowering agents, and psychotropic drugs. *Semin Liver Dis*. 2002;22:169–183.
242. Tolman KG. The liver and lovastatin. *Am J Cardiol*. 2002;89:1374–1380.
243. Pasternak RC, Smith SC, Bairey-Merz CN, Grundy SM, Cleman JI, Lenfant C. ACC/AHA/NHLBI clinical advisory on the use and safety of statins. *J Am Coll Cardiol*. 2002;40:567–572.
244. Robert WC. Getting more people on statins. *Am J Cardiol*. 2002;90:683–685.
245. Cohen DE, Anania FA, Chalasani N. An assessment of statin safety by hepatologists. *Am J Cardiol*. 2006;97(suppl):77C–81C.
246. McKenney JM, Davidson MH, Jacobson TA, Guyton JR. Final conclusions and recommendations of the National Lipid Association Statin Safety Assessment Task Force. *Am J Cardiol*. 2006;97(suppl):89C–94C.
247. Guthrie RM, Martin DR. The safety of rosuvastatin: effects on renal and hepatic function. *Expert Opin Drug Saf*. 2007;6:573–581.
248. US Food and Drug Administration. FDA Drug alert: Rosuvastatin. March 11, 2005. http://www.fda.gov/cder/drug/infopage/rosuvastatin/default.htm. Accessed January 22, 2009.
249. Sidaway JE, Davidson RG, Taggart F, et al. Inhibitors of 3-hydroxy-3-methylglutaryl-CoA-reductase reduce receptor-mediated endocytosis in opossum kidney cells. *J Am Soc Nephrol*. 2004;15:2258–2265.
250. Verhulst A, D'Haese PCD, DeBroe ME. Inhibitors of HMG-CoA reductase reduce receptor-mediated endocytosis in human kidney proximal tubular cells. *J Am Soc Nephrol*. 2004;15:2249–2257.
251. Agarwal R. Statin induced proteinuria: renal injury or renoprotection? *J Am Soc Nephrol*. 2004;15:2502–2503.
252. Tonolo G, Ciccarese M, Brizzi P, et al. Reduction of albumin excretion rate in normotensive microalbuminuric type 2 diabetic patients during long-term simvastatin treatment. *Diabetes Care*. 1997;20:1891–1895.
253. Lee TM, Su SF, Tsai CH. Effect of pravastatin on proteinuria in patients with well-controlled hypertension. *Hypertension*. 2002;40:67–73.
254. Bianchi S, Bigazzi R, Caiazza A, Campese VM. A controlled prospective study of the effects of atorvastatin on proteinuria and progression of kidney disease. *Am J Kidney Dis*. 2003;41:565–570.
255. Tonelli M, Moye L, Sacks FM, et al; Cholesterol and Recurrent Event (CARE) Trial Investigators. Effect of pravastatin on loss of renal function in people with moderate chronic renal insufficiency and cardiovascular disease. *J Am Soc Nephrol*. 2003;14:1605–1613.
256. Fried LF, Orchard TJ, Kasiske BL; Lipids and Renal Disease Progression Meta-Analysis Study Group. Effect of lipid reduction on the progression of renal disease: a meta-analysis. *Kidney Int*. 2001;59:260–269.
257. Vidt DG, Cressman MD, Harris S, Pears JS, Hutchinson HG. Rosuvastatin-induced arrest in progression of renal disease. *Cardiology*. 2004;102:52–60.
258. Zetia [package insert]. North Wales, PA: Merck/Schering-Plough; 2007.
259. Vytorin [package insert]. North Wales, PA: Merck/Schering-Plough; 2007.
260. Jackevicius CA, Jack JV, Tu JV, Ross JS, Ko DT, Krumholz HM. Use of ezetimibe in the United States and Canada. *N Engl J Med*. 2008;358:1819–1828.
261. Kastelein JJP, Akdim FF, Stroes ESG, et al. Simvastatin with or without ezetimibe in familial hypercholesterolemia. *N Engl J Med*. 2008;358:1431–1443.
262. Brown BG, Taylor AJ. Does ENHANCE diminish confidence in lowering LDL or in ezetimibe? *N Engl J Med*. 2008;358:1504–1507.
263. Drazen JM, Jarcho JA, Morrissey S, Curfman GD. Cholesterol lowering and ezetimibe. *N Engl J Med*. 2008;358:1507–1508.
264. Rossebo AB, Pedersen TR, Boman K, et al. Intensive lipid lowering with simvastatin and ezetimibe in Aortic Stenosis. *N Engl J Med*. 2008;359:1343–1355.

265. Peto R, Emberson J, Landray M, et al. Analyses of cancer data from three ezetimibe trials. *N Engl J Med*. 2008;359:1357–1366.
266. O'Riordan M. Ezetimibe controversy continues: IMPROVE-IT enlarged and delayed, then inside struggle over ENHANCE. *Heartwire*. March 31, 2008. http://www.theheart.org/article/852455.do. Accessed January 22, 2009.
267. Tenkanen L, Manttari M, Kovaanen PT, Virkunen H, Manninen V. Gemfibrozil in the treatment of dyslipidemia. An 18-year mortality follow-up of the Helsinki Heart Study. *Arch Intern Med*. 2006;166:743–748.
268. The FIELD Study Investigators. Effects of long-term fenofibrate therapy on cardiovascular events in 9795 people with type 2 diabetes mellitus (the FIELD study): randomised controlled trial. *Lancet*. 2005;366:1849–1861.
269. The BIP Study Group. Secondary Prevention by raising HDL cholesterol and reducing triglycerides in patients with coronary artery disease. The Benzafibrate Infarction Prevention (BIP) Study. *Circulation*. 2000;102:21–27.
270. Ginsberg HN, Bonds DE, Lovato LC, et al. Evolution of the lipid trial protocol of the Action to Control Cardiovascular Risk in Diabetes (ACCORD) Trial. *Am J Cardiol*. 2007;99(suppl):56i–67i.
271. Davidson MH, Carlson DM, Guthrie RM, et al. ABT-335 in combination with rosuvastatin improves multiple lipid ratios in patients with mixed dyslipidemia. *J Clin Lipidol*. 2008;2:211–212.
272. Tricor [package insert]. North Chicago, IL: Abbott Laboratories; 2004.
273. Cannere PL, Berge KG, Wengler NK, et al. Fifteen year mortality in Coronary Drug Project patients: long-term benefit with niacin. *J Am Coll Cardiol*. 1986;8:1245–1255.
274. Brown BG, Zhao XQ, Chait A, et al. Simvastatin and niacin, antioxidant vitamins, or the combination for the prevention of coronary disease. *N Engl J Med*. 2001;345:1583–1592.
275. Blankenhorn DH, Nessim SA, Johnson RL, Sanmarco ME, Azen SP, Cashin-Hemphill L. Beneficial effects of combined colestipol-niacin therapy on coronary atherosclerosis and coronary bypass grafts. *JAMA*. 1987;257:3233–3240.
276. Cashin-Hemphill L, Mack WJ, Pogoda JM, Sanmarco ME, Azen SP, Blankenhorn DH. Beneficial effects of colestipol-niacin on coronary atherosclerosis. A 4-year follow-up. *JAMA*. 1990;264: 3013–3017.
277. Carlson LA, Rosenhameera G. Reduction of mortality in the Stockholm Ischaemic Heart Disease Secondary Prevention Study by combined treatment with clofibrate and nicotinic acid. *Acta Med Scand*. 1988;223:405–418.
278. AIM-HIGH: Niacin plus statin to prevent vascular events. ClinicalTrials.gov Website. http://clinicaltrials.gov/ct2/show/NCT00120289. Updated December 29, 2008. Accessed January 22, 2009.
279. Niaspan [package insert]. Miami, FL: KOS Pharmaceuticals; 2004.
280. Grundy SM, Vega GL, McGovern, et al. Efficacy, safety and tolerability of once-daily niacin for the treatment of dyslipidemia associated with type 2 diabetes. *Arch Intern Med*. 2002;162: 1568–1576.
281. Carlson LA. Nicotinic acid: the broad-spectrum lipid drug. A 50th anniversary review. *J Intern Med*. 2005;258:94–114.
282. LaRosa J. Review of clinical studies of bile acid sequestrants for lowering plasma lipid levels. *Cardiology*. 1989;76(suppl 1):55–64.
283. Cholestyramine. In: *The Complete Drug Reference at Micromedex Healthcare Series*. London, UK: Pharmaceutical Press; 2008.
284. Colestipol Hydrochloride. In: *The Complete Drug Reference at Micromedex Healthcare Series* (Internet database). Greenwood Village, CO: Thomson Healthcare. Updated periodically.
285. Welchol [package insert]. Parsippany, NJ: Daiichi-Sankyo Pharmaceuticals; 2006.
286. Blankenhorn DH, Nessim SA, Johnson RL, Sanmarco ME, Azen SP, Cashin-Hemphill L. Beneficial effects of combined colestipol-niacin therapy on coronary atherosclerosis and coronary venous bypass grafts. *JAMA*. 1987;257:3013–3017.
287. Kane JP, Malloy MJ, Phillips NR, Phillips NR, Diehl JC, Havel RJ. Regression of coronary atherosclerosis during treatment of familial hypercholesterolemia with combined drug regimens. *JAMA*. 1990;264:3007–3012.
288. Marchioli R, Barzi F, Bomba E, et al. Early protection against sudden death by n-3 polyunsaturated fatty acids after myocardial infarction. *Circulation*. 2002;105:1897–1903.
289. Leaf A, Albert CM, Josephenson M, et al. Prevention of fatal arrhythmias in high-risk subjects by fish oil n-3 fatty acid intake. *Circulation*. 2005;112:2762–2768.
290. Brouwer IA, Zock PL, Camm AJ, et al. Effect of fish oil on ventricular tachyarrhythmia and

death in patients with implantable cardioverter defibrillators. *JAMA*. 2006;295:2613–2619.
291. Riatt MH, Connor WE, Morris C, et al. Fish oil supplementation and risk of ventricular tachycardia and ventricular fibrillation in patients with implantable defibrillators. *JAMA*. 2005;293:2884–2891.
292. Lovaza [package insert]. Liberty Corner, NJ: Reliant Pharmaceuticals; 2007.
293. Rader D. Illuminating HDL—is it still a viable therapeutic target? *N Engl J Med*. 2007;357: 2180–2183.
294. Tall A, Yvan-Charvet L, Wang N. The failure of torcetrapib: was it the molecule or the mechanism? *Arterioscler Thromb Vasc Biol*. 2007;27:257–260.
295. Kastelein JJP, van Leuven SI, Burgess L, et al. Effect of torcetrapib on carotid atherosclerosis in familial hypercholesterolemia. *N Engl J Med*. 2007;356:1620–1630.
296. Nissen SE, Tardif JC, Nicholls SJ, et al. Effect of torcetrapib on the progression of coronary atherosclerosis. *N Engl J Med*. 2007;356:1304–1316.
297. Krumholz HM, Lee TH. Redefining quality—implications of recent clinical trials. *N Engl J Med*. 2008;358:2537–2539.
298. Tall AR. CETP inhibitors to increase HDL cholesterol levels. *N Engl J Med*. 2007;356:1364–1366.
299. Young JM, Florkowski CM, Molyneux SL, et al. Effect of coenzyme Q_{10} supplementation on simvastatin-induced myalgia. *Am J Cardio*. 2007; 100:1400–1403.
300. Caso G, Kelly P, McNurlan MA, Lawson WE. Effect of coenzyme Q_{10} in myopathic symptoms in patients treated with statins. *Am J Cardiol*. 2007; 99:1409–1412.

INDEX